INTERMITTENT FASTING FOR WOMEN OVER 50

Purify your Body while Losing Weight and Increasing Energy

Author

Mildred E. Howard

Table of Contents

BONUS INTERMITTENT FASTING RECIPES

CHAPTER 18: COOKING TIPS

CHAPTER 19: FREQUENTLY ASKED QUESTIONS (FAQS)

CONCLUSION

Introduction

Dieting is difficult! There are such a large number of alternatives available that occasionally it can feel overwhelming – you find yourself in a situation where you don't know where to start from. Or then again, perhaps you've attempted them all – the gluten-free diet, the Atkins diet, the Paleo diet – and none of them was able to help you, so you need to try something new. This is where intermittent fasting comes in. It's one of the best approaches to get in shape, and for an excellent reason: this is not a diet; in fact, it deals with the way you eat. It's a method for planning your meals, so take advantage of them. There is an incredible number of benefits in picking this technique, including the one of getting more fit and getting rid of stomach fat. It can improve your overall wellbeing – assisting in resolving conditions like diabetes and heart issues. It can likewise assist you in living without diseases, serving as help long-term. It's of great advantage to your brain, and it can really assist you with living longer.

Intermittent Fasting for women over 50 may help reduce breast cancer risk, according to a study published in the journal Cancer Research. Intermittent Fasting is becoming more popular as the years go on. While most people are familiar with this for men, women over 50 can benefit from it too. This kind of Fasting is a dieting technique that involves short periods of fasting every day. It has become increasingly popular as a weight-loss method for women over the age of 50.

Intermittent Fasting is a diet that allows you to eat all the food you want during a specific fasting window. It can help you lose weight. However, this kind of Fasting is more than just losing weight. Intermittent Fasting for women over 50 is all about eating fewer calories while still nourishing your body. During the fasting period, you'll eat 500 calories on non-fasting days and 1,000 calories on fasting days.

Intermittent Fasting is when you restrict calories or eating hours during the week. It is the opposite of what we usually do, which is to eat a certain amount every day of the week (a diet). This is frequently referred to as "caloric restriction", and it has been shown to prolong life in many research studies.

When you restrict your calories, such as when you fast, your body is forced to use more of its own fat for energy. This is not captured by most people because they are in a calorie deficit and thus not eating enough to give their bodies the energy needed. The caloric restriction is part of intermittent Fasting as opposed to dieting, where calorie restriction is only one part of the equation.

Intermittent Fasting (IF) can sound very restrictive, but there are many strategies and plans out there to help you make it easier to do. For example, you can switch from eating breakfast every day to fasting breakfast every day, or you can just start by skipping dinner on a specific day each week. The main reason why this diet is successful is that it lowers the concentration of fat in your body, as well as the number of calories you eat.

Chapter 1: What is Intermittent Fasting

Intermittent Fasting is a regimen of controlled meal placement and controlled periods of Fasting. At first glance, it may simply look like meal skipping, but the added element that can't be missed or forgotten is ensuring that our bodies are getting the nourishment they require throughout each day, even on the days when we've chosen not to eat anything. The core concept of intermittent Fasting doesn't dictate what you should or should not be eating, but it does dictate the intervals at which you eat and at which you fast.

With intermittent fasting, you're cutting down your calorie intake by shaving off a meal here and there throughout your week, and you're giving your body the chance to adapt and boost its hormone production that will allow you to access and break down those stores of fat your body has created over the years. By doing this, you'll find that your body is creating energy, even when you have not eaten recently.

Because your body will be getting accustomed to this method of living and this means of procuring energy, you'll find that you have more energy on a more consistent basis throughout the day. Because your body has onboard stores of energy that it can now access, you won't experience those midday slumps or crashes. You won't feel faint after several hours of not eating because your body is still getting everything it needs from those stores!

Stages of Intermittent Fasting

• After 12 hours of Fasting, the body has reached the metabolic stage ofketosis. The body continues to burn and break down fat in this condition.

• After 18 hours, the body has moved to the fat-burning mode and producesessential ketones.

• After 24 hours, the body's cells gradually replace old components andbreak down defective proteins associated with Alzheimer's and other neurodegenerative diseases. This is a strategy called autophagy.

For tissue and cell rejuvenation, autophagy is an essential mechanism that eliminates weakened cellular components, including defected proteins. Severe consequences happen when the cells don't or can't activate autophagy, like many neurodegenerative disorders, which tend to develop due to diminished autophagy during ageing.

• After 48 hours, the body's growth hormone output is up by five times asstrong, without consuming calories or with very little calories, carbohydrates, or protein when one begins their fast.

This process explains that ketone bodies formed throughout Fasting can facilitate growth hormone secretion in the brain. Ghrelin, the starvation hormone, often promotes development hormone secretion. Growth hormone helps maintain lean muscle mass, particularly as we mature, and it decreases the buildup of fat tissue. It also tends to play a part in humans' survival and may facilitate cardiovascular wellbeing and wound healing.

• After 54 hours, insulin has fallen to its lowest amount after a person hasbegun fasting, and the body gets more and more insulin-sensitive. Decreased amounts of insulin provide a variety of long-term and short-term health effects.

• After 72 hours, the body breaks down aged immune cells and creates newones.

• Intermittent Fasting can also influence risk factors, such as blood sugarlevels and reducing cholesterol, for health problems such as cardiovascular disease and diabetes.

During Fasting, the cells often perform important repair mechanisms, which alter the expression of genes. One can lose weight with Intermittent Fasting, as it also impacts hormones. It's because it is the way the body processes body fat as energy calories. The body makes many improvements when you do not consume something and makes the accumulated energy more usable.

Examples involve shifts in the nervous system's function and drastic changes in certain essential hormones' quantities.

Two metabolic modifications mentioned below occur when a person fasts:

• Insulin: When a person consumes food, insulin levels rise, and whenFasting begins, they decline drastically. Fat burning is encouraged by reduced amounts of insulin.

• Norepinephrine or Noradrenaline: Norepinephrine is forwarded to the fatcells by the nervous system, allowing them to disintegrate body fat into unsaturated fatty acids that can be used for energy.

Here are several alterations that occur while fasting in the human body:

• (HGH)Human Growth Hormone: Growth hormone levels riseexponentially by as many as five times. This has muscle gain and fat loss advantages as well as many others.

• Insulin: Sensitivity to insulin increases, and insulin levels decreasesignificantly. Low levels of insulin improve the ability of the body to use stored fat.

• Cellular repair: The cells begin cellular repair while fasting. This meansautophagy, where aged and damaged proteins build up within cells, digest, and kill unhealthy cells.

• Gene expression: There are improvements in longevity-related geneexpression and defence against disease.

Intermittent Fasting's health benefits can be seen as these variations in hormone levels, cell structure, and gene expression occur.

Chapter 2: The science of IF (what is autophagy, how it works, etc.)

Like any thought of eating that rapidly assumes control over the wellbeing and diet societies, Intermittent Fasting has been suspected to be a craze. In any case, the proof behind Fasting's points of interest is as of now clear—and expanding.

There are a few theories concerning why intermittent Fasting performs so well. However, the strain has to do with the most generally examined—and most demonstrated addition.

The term pressure has been denounced persistently; however, the body benefits from some pressure. Exercise, for instance, is, in fact, weight on the body (particularly on the muscles and the cardiovascular framework). In any case, this particular pressure, at last, improves the body as long as you execute the right measure of recuperation period into your activity plan.

Intermittent Fasting stresses the body similarly to that activity does; it brings the phones under moderate strain as you decline the body nourishment for a specific period. Cells react to this strain over the long haul by concentrating on how to more readily adapt to it. It has an improved capacity to oppose sickness on the grounds that the body turns out to be better at managing torment.

Autophagy is an essential cycle where the body's cells "clear out" any unnecessary or damaged segments. Fasting and calorie limitation puts the body's cells under pressure. At the point when an individual restricts the amount of food that goes into their body, their cells get fewer calories than they need to work effectively.

When this occurs, the cells should work all the more effectively. Because of the pressure welcomed by Fasting or calorie limitation, autophagy makes the body's cells clear out and reuse any pointless or damaged components.

Autophagy: Nature's Detoxifier

Now that you are aware of the processes behind autophagy, we will discuss autophagy's cleaning capabilities. The science behind it makes intermittent Fasting better than other strategies to increase your health, ending up doing more harm than good. It tells us that it is something that all of us should be thinking about — even if we are not trying to lose weight — because it just has that much influence on our bodies.

You can be promised that you haven't discovered all that this dietary supplement can do for your body until you begin to take it regularly. In my experience, there's quite a lot of proof that kale is a superfood that is very good for health because it is packed with so many vitamins and nutrients that your body requires.

Some people misinterpret scientific evidence in order to make it seem as though kale is the only nutritious food to eat. They advocate diets that mix kale with other foods during the day. Of course, eating more kale is good for you, but it will still not be as effective as bringing about autophagy. That's because although eating vegetables is crucial for wellness, it doesn't provide everything you need, and most importantly, it doesn't actually make you whole.

On the other hand, autophagy is highly important to your body. It's a process that happens to you whether you like it or not; even if you never think about it, it will always happen to you. If cells do not go through it, they die, and the human being dies with them. This is what distinguishes detoxifying your body with something like kale and detoxifying with autophagy. We are talking about what the body already does and how to make it even better than before.

Even though people might feel like they're using more energy, their cells are still in use of more. Unlike you and me, they do not have the luxury of sleep or energy to heal. This is what makes autophagy a central part of a cell's functions: when you fast and your cells' food supplies are exhausted, they still need the energy to keep on going — so they find their energy in the nooks and crannies. Your cells absorb unused proteins, broken down fats, and autophagosomes start working extra hard to recognize toxins found in your body. They are extra motivated to do this when you fast because cells need to work to survive.

Our cells don't care about their state of cleanliness the way we do. You only care about their cleanliness because they work much efficiently when they have cleared out the toxins, and that's where all the positive health effects of autophagy come from. But since your cells don't care for themselves, they will let things get very crowded: they will have toxins all over and will simply die off when it becomes so much that they can't work properly.

Of course, they will eventually go through some maintenance mode when you go to sleep. Therefore, you are reading this book because you want the cells to go beyond the cells' usual capacities to optimize health outcomes.

We're letting our cellular bodies breakdown in the modern-day. After your first intermittent Fasting, you'll see how much we eat every day without realizing it. To briefly look at things from a philosophical standpoint, we continually load ourselves with so many things, and we don't give ourselves a chance to clean ourselves out. Autophagy comes in as the last option. Our bodies are not prepared to handle the amount of junk we eat today, so we have to think about our cells proactively to make sure they are doing their job.

Everyone knows about the contaminants that we are exposed to in this modern day. If we don't regularly practice intermittent Fasting, some of these can affect our long-term health with negative consequences. I do not recommend being paranoid about the chemicals in our foods. Nevertheless, it is a fact that our foods are packed with them, and it is difficult to be completely positive that all of them are fine for us. We may not be able to remove these chemicals from our atmosphere fully, but we can get rid of the ones that do end up in our bodies through the natural process of autophagy.

This process will not only leave you having a clean system that will reduce your exposure to various harmful toxins, but you will also feel better. You can really feel the difference subjectively. We briefly discuss the physical health side of things, but because of this, we must also discuss the emotional part. It's reassuring to know that one's body is consistently removing toxins, which can bring relief during difficult times—using IF involves not only improving your physical health as much as possible but also spending time improving your psychological health.

When the detox is a big part of what you want autophagy to do for you, you may be motivated to make it as potent as possible by using a variety of triggering methods, IF should be your main method of triggering autophagy since it is the easiest, and therefore, the most reliable. But once you start feeling the difference in your skin and under it — once the work your cells are doing is a sensation you detect throughout your biological systems, there are extremely high chances that you will get emotionally addicted to it and want more. You can combine intermittent Fasting with many other methods to yield even greater detoxification. If you live anywhere where you have saunas available, it will be advantageous. Saunas do so much good for your body, as they can make your heart rate go down, increase the circulation of your blood, and do a detox on your body directly through your skin. Saunas apply tension to the body to get your cells in shape. If you remember, autophagy is the thing that causes cells to shift into a state of stress. Fasting, or intermittent fasting, is the easiest way to simulate the normal stress response, but saunas may be helpful as well.

And if you don't have a real sauna, you can still reap some benefits from taking a hot shower, as the steam can permeate into your skin and help detoxify your body. Therefore, the cells will release some of the stress associated with sauna therapy. Implementing a sauna or hot shower in place of intermittent Fasting is not the best way to maximize autophagy and shouldn't be recommended. However, if you use intermittent Fasting alongside such techniques, autophagy will be increased.

What Is The Relationship Between Intermittent Fasting And Autophagy?

Autophagy can use old cell parts and recycle them to create new energy that the organism (like the human or animal) can use to do its regular functions like walking and breathing.

People are now studying what happens when humans rely on this form of energy production instead of the energy they would get from ingesting food throughout the day. This point is where Autophagy and Intermittent Fasting come together. We will delve deeply into intermittent Fasting and Autophagy and how they work together to allow for things like weight loss or disease prevention.

Scientists who have been studying this for some time are not beginning to understand that there are ways to manipulate the process of Autophagy within the human body to achieve weight loss, improved health, reduction of disease symptoms, and so on.

The most common way to induce Autophagy in a person is by way of starvation. This kind of starvation is not to say that a person must starve themselves, but they starve their cells of nutrition temporarily. This benefit is why people turn to fast to induce Autophagy.

Low nutrition levels within the cells are the most common way that Autophagy is triggered, as it is a process that creates energy within the cell. By knowing this, scientists have concluded that by inducing starvation within the cells, one can intentionally upregulate Autophagy in one body. Intermittent Fasting involves fasting periods, which then induces a state of starvation within the cells (simply meaning that there is no energy being consumed to use for energy). So it induces Autophagy in the cells to make energy.

Other Ways To Induce Autophagy

Along with Intermittent Fasting, there are other ways that you can encourage the cells of your body to use Autophagy to their fullest potential. Below is a list of these other methods. They will help you understand how to make the most of the benefits of intermittent Fasting and Autophagy in your body.

Cell Starvation

The most common way to induce Autophagy in a person is by way of starvation. Autophagy is triggered by a decrease in nutrients within a cell. As I mentioned above, this decrease in nutrients acts as a signal within the cell to begin Autophagy, which is exactly how Intermittent Fasting works.

Aerobic Exercise

One other way to activate Autophagy is through exercise. Aerobic exercise has been shown through studies to increase Autophagy in the cells of the muscles, the heart, the brain, lungs, and the liver.

Sleep

Sleep is very important for Autophagy. If you have ever gone a few days without proper, restful sleep, you know that you begin to feel a decline in your mental abilities rather quickly. This effect could be because of your brain's decreased autophagy functioning. The number of hours you are in bed does not matter if the sleep is not of good quality.

Quality sleep for the right number of hours is needed to maintain good brain function and keep your brain's Autophagy going.

Consuming Specific Foods

The consumption of specific foods has been shown to induce or promote Autophagy. The added benefit is that not only do they trigger Autophagy in the cells of your body, these foods are also shown to have numerous other health benefits.

Autophagy and Your Skin

Now that you know all about the science of how IF impacts your skin, we will go deeper into how IF can effectively treat your skin.

First of all, it's important to realize the importance of hydration to the skin. You may be going through autophagy 12 hours a day, but that won't necessarily help your skin condition. Many people do not get enough water intake per day. You should drink seven glasses of water at least every day. It is clear this is the most important step that can be taken for your skin. Earlier, you learned how the two mechanisms detoxify your system. Well, this means that your pores are cleared out, too. No one wants to keep their pores clogged, and if you drink plenty of water and keep up your habit of intermittent fasting, you won't have to worry about clogged pores in your skin for much longer.

The way that IF helps boost your skin is in two ways. For one, autophagy cleans away the toxic build-up that obstructs the pores. But it also assists you in developing healthy skin cells. This results in the long-term result and more desired effect of more elastic and more youthful skin.

When you keep your skin healthy with autophagy, your true goal is to increase the amount of collagen your skin cells produce.

It is actually not all of your skin cells that produce the collagen protein, but just some of them. These skin cells are called fibroblasts. Fibroblasts are specialized cells made to produce the protein we have been talking about, known as collagen.

You cannot go wrong with collagen — the more you have in your body, the healthier and more elastic your skin becomes. Though we may be 18 years old, our fibroblasts usually produce less collagen and the rate at which our skin can stretch decreases. If you wish to develop new collagen, you must ensure your cells are in good health by drinking plenty of water and undergoing Intermittent Fasting. Our fibroblasts avoid producing collagen because they get clogged with toxins, similar to occlusive damage in our pores. Cells show less overall proliferation because toxins outnumber them. The unused proteins, organelles, and other toxins accumulate, whereby they can eventually cause cellular damage.

When we say that autophagy helps your skin in two ways, it means that one way causes the other to clean out your pores, and in turn, this makes your fibroblasts healthier and more successful. Better cells can do their job better, and skin cells get tighter as a result.

One important purpose of skincare is for looking good; however, it also includes keeping skin safe. Your skin is the most essential of your many organs. Good skin protects against various skin cancers, ultraviolet rays, and diseases, making their spread to the skin's cells.

The skin cells of your skin organ are a perfect example in general because skin cells continue to get replaced over the month. The mechanism of autophagy is important to the continual renewal of the skin cells. Triggering the supplement with IF would result in health benefits because you protect the continuous natural cycle of skin cells you need.

When detoxifying the body, the skin is the best way to get rid of toxins. It is your first line of protection against contaminants that you come in contact with through the environment.

It is also the best way to get better, healthier skin because it can tackle this continual cycle of new cells in your skin. No other method can deal with the constant stream of new skin cells, which is why they tend to fail.

For instance, there are endless skincare products that claim to do what autophagy does for your skin, but this is impossible since these products can't compete with how it goes deep into your layers of skin, to your old cells and new cells.

These skincare products can only put creme on top of your outermost layer of skin, making it look better, but it is only covering it up without solving the problem that can only be solved through cellular means.

Regrettably, so many people spend time and money on unsuccessful goods, but at least you won't have to. In fact, the improved health and youthfulness of your skin will probably be the first thing you notice as a result of Intermittent Fasting. Along with weight loss, it is commonly reported as the first noticeable difference.

The urge to lose weight and to have better-looking skin always go hand in hand. One explanation for this is fear of the so-called "skin curtain." As we said before, loose skin from weight loss has a lot of variables that go into it: (1) the pace at which you lose the weight, (2) how much weight is lost, (3) genetics, (4) age, and (5) the health of your skin. Not only can we deal with loose skin later in life, but many of these problems can also be avoided in the first place. We influence them. Let's get started with loose skin regulation once you have it.

People shouldn't worry about loose skin from weight loss because it doesn't affect the body permanently. Of course, these things often go on a case-bycase basis, so most people looking at loose skin after weight loss don't have to allow it into their lives. Numerous options exist for how to treat it after the operation; surgery isn't the only option. Working to minimize loose skin is equivalent to preserving healthy skin in general. You want to drink seven to eight glasses of water per day and still have the recommended amount of physical activity.

Getting rid of loose skin will take time, but it is simpler than extra fat on your body. It is remarkable how many people fear losing weight due to their unfounded fear of loose skin, do not let yourself be one of them. And people can control loose skin until they lose weight. It is not permanent; it is just like being overweight or obese is just temporary. Much like the qualities mentioned above, you just have to regularly put in the effort and be patient as time can help tighten loose skin after weight loss.

You may reduce the risk of developing loose skin in the first place, too. Your age and how much weight you want to lose are not things that you can control, but you can control other things: how much water you drink and how soon you lose the weight, whether you get enough nutrients, and whether you exercise.

Most importantly, you can do the first method to trigger the other, which will help with loose skin the most. Research shows that people who fast deal with less loose skin when they lose the weight they want to lose. Take care of the things you can control, and if you still have some loose skin when the weight is off, keep taking care of your body, and following your IF routine, so your skin tightens as quickly as possible.

You may use the experience of fasting to hold loose skin at bay in the future. Many people assume that their skin becomes dry when they go on a long-term fast and starts to crack. You can feel this slightly without thinking about it, but if the feeling goes further than that, you may want to stop your quick early. You are still not adapting to your new body shape well enough, and if you continue at your current rate, you will have loose skin that you don't want.

Your skin is the organ that people can see, and this is the reason why there is a multi-million-dollar industry around skincare products. Regardless of how the skin looks, beauty should not be a primary concern. People should also want to lose weight to look healthier, but this does not come at the cost of their wellbeing. Women need to keep track of their skin health because sometimes they use so many products that they are unsure of their skin health's natural state.

After you take a shower, examine your skin and consider the state. Regularly checking your skin will keep you motivated to exercise more. You'll notice dramatic improvements easily. Your skin's primary function is not to draw attention but to shield the body from contaminants on the outer surface. You are doing IF will allow you to protect your skin against pathogens and microbes. With good treatment, the skin will look better as well. It is a win-win scenario.

A continuous daily supply of food requires a significant effort by your digestive system to process, digest, and absorb the nutrients of the food you eat. The brain centres that regulate appetite in some people are not good at constantly monitoring daily food intake effectively. Our body has several defence mechanisms to prevent starvation and nutritional deficiencies, and one of them is hunger. Although this was a great tool for ancient hunters and gatherers, it is less useful today when food is available. Therefore, obesity and its health consequences are increasingly common in the modern population. Choosing intermittent Fasting, which serves as a diet for losing weight, can be a natural way to adjust your diet and its effectiveness in controlling your weight and protecting you from hearing damage and high cholesterol. Intermittent Fasting works through several mechanisms that help maintain normal body weight and health:
Appetite Control

Intermittent Fasting encourages the body to use parts of the diet more efficiently and prevents excessive accumulation of fat. When we eat more calories than we consume through physical and mental work, our body will store excess energy in the form of fat deposits. As a protective mechanism against hunger and malnutrition, which developed when our ancestors struggled to eat, our appetite is not a great means of regulating our diet, as it will always make us eat more than we really need. Our appetite, which is located in the lower centres of the brain that are not under the control of the higher regions of the brain responsible for logic and reasoning, we cannot know how much work and mental muscle will do after eating. Intermittent Fasting allows our body to adjust to temporary food shortages and use food more efficiently without storing fat.

Improved Metabolism

During the short-term lack of food, energy consumption increases by a higher level of adrenaline in the blood (also known as epinephrine), as shown in the medical research from 2000 at the University in Vienna, Austria, and published in the American Journal of Clinical Nutrition. It is an adaptive mechanism that causes the mobilization of fat reserves and the accelerated burning of carbohydrates and fatty acids. The result is an improved metabolism that will lead to gradual weight loss unless you do not eat unhealthy foods on your non-fasting days.

Intermittent Fasting works similarly with fiscal moderation, which also causes an increase in blood adrenaline levels and greater weight loss.

Calorie Reduction
Intermittent Fasting is associated with a reduction of calories. If you do not eat large amounts of food on non-fasting days, the diet will reduce the number of calories. However, unlike the daily calorie limit, intermittent

Fasting allows you to eat some of your favourite foods for days without fasting. In addition to reducing calorie intake, Intermittent Fasting offers other important health benefits, such as accelerated removal of toxic substances from the digestive system, improved metabolism, improved blood circulation, and even longevity.

Chapter 3: Myths around IF

Fasting has become increasingly common.

One ongoing misconception is that breakfast is the most vital meal of the day.

People also assume that missing breakfast contributes to intense hunger, cravings, and weight gain.

One 16-week survey in 283 overweight and obese adults showed little difference in weight between those who ate breakfast and those who did not.

Thus, the weight is not largely affected by breakfast, although there may be some individual variability. Some research also suggests that people who lose weight in the long term prefer to eat breakfast.

Moreover, children and teens who eat breakfast tend to do better in school.

As such, you are paying attention to your particular needs is crucial. Breakfast is beneficial for certain individuals, while others may miss it without any negative consequences.

Breakfast can help a lot of people, but it is not essential for your health. Regulated studies do not indicate any difference in weight loss between those who eat breakfast and those who miss it

Eating frequently boosts your metabolism

Many people assume that your metabolic rate is boosted by consuming more meals, allowing your body to consume more calories overall.

Indeed, the body spends some calories digesting meals.
On average, about 10 per cent of the total calorie intake is used by TEF.

What matters, however, is the overall amount of calories you consume, not how many meals you eat.

Consuming six 500-calorie meals has the same impact as eating three meals with 1,000 calories. Provided an average TEF of 10 per cent, you will burn 300 calories in both cases.

Numerous studies indicate that increasing or reducing the duration of meals does not affect overall calories burned.

Contrary to common opinion, eating smaller meals frequently doesn't increase your metabolism.

Eating frequently also helps reduce hunger.

Some people think that eating regularly helps to reduce cravings and excessive hunger.

Yet, the evidence is mixed.

While some studies indicate that consuming more regular meals results in decreased hunger, other studies have found little impact or even increased levels of hunger.

One research compared three or six high protein meals a day showed that consuming three meals decreased hunger more effectively than eating three meals.

That said, responses may be dependent on the individual. If regular eating decreases your cravings, it's probably a good idea. Still, there is no proof that eating or snacking more frequently decreases hunger for everyone.

Intermittent Fasting makes you lose muscle
Some people claim that your body starts burning muscles for fuel when you fast.

Though this happens in general with dieting, no evidence indicates that it occurs more with intermittent Fasting than other methods.

On the other hand, studies show that intermittent fasting is better for mass muscle maintenance.

In one study, intermittent fasting resulted in a comparable amount of weight loss as continuous calorie limitation but with much less muscle mass reduction.

Another research showed a small increase in muscle mass for individuals who ate all their calories during a large evening meal. Although you may have heard rumours that intermittent Fasting affects your health, studies show that it has many outstanding health benefits.

For instance, it alters the gene expression associated with longevity and immunity and has been shown to extend the lifespan of animals.

It also has important metabolic health benefits, such as increased insulin sensitivity and reduced oxidative stress, heart disease, and inflammation.

It may also enhance brain wellbeing by increasing levels of brain-derived neurotrophic factor (BDNF), a hormone that can defend against depression and many other psychiatric disorders.

Intermittent Fasting makes you overeat

Some people claim that intermittent Fasting makes you overeat during eating periods.

Although it is true you may compensate for calories lost during a fast by automatically eating a little more afterwards, this compensation is not complete.

One research found that individuals who fasted for 24 hours actually ended up eating about 500 extra calories the next day, far less than the 2,400 calories they lost during the fast.

Because it decreases total food intake and insulin levels while increasing metabolism, human growth hormone (HGH) levels, and norepinephrine levels, intermittent Fasting makes you lose fat — not gain it

According to one study, Fasting for 3-24 weeks led to average weight and belly fat losses of 3-8 per cent and 4-7 per cent, respectively.

As such, one of the most effective methods for losing weight might be intermittent Fasting.

Fasting Decreases Your Metabolism

Some individuals worry that Fasting decreases your resting metabolic rate (in other words, Fasting makes you burn fewer calories at rest). The fear is that you'll put on weight like a three-toed sloth when you start eating normally again.

This is what happens on diets that limit calories, which include eating 50 to 85 per cent of the food your body needs on a long-term daily basis. Your metabolism adapts to the lower consumption of energy, and it can remain that way for years.

You Shouldn't Drink Water While Fasting.

Some religious fasts include both the restriction of food and water, such as Ramadan fasting. Possibly unrelated, a variety of rumours that no-water fasts are optimal for health have emerged.

Sadly, because Fasting has a diuretic effect, water restriction can lead to unsafe dehydration. That's why when supervising patients undertaking therapeutic fasts, doctors pay careful attention to fluid intake. Physicians often pay careful attention to electrolytes, such as potassium and sodium, both of which are energetically peed out during Fasting.

You Can't Gain Muscle While Fasting.

Fasting doesn't seem to be the right way for muscle building. You don't need to pound protein shakes after all?

Well, protein is what you need, but you don't need it 24/7. For example, active women practising 16/8 fasting acquired just as much muscle and strength in one 2019 study as women eating on a more traditional schedule.

Here is the thing. In times of scarcity, the body works hard to preserve muscle.

Think of it this way: our ancestors would have been too weak to hunt if humans burned through muscles during a fast!

Fasting Makes You Overindulge

You'll be hungry after a fast. This hunger, many believe, will cause subsequent overeating.

It's For Everyone

Intermittent Fasting is very popular right now. It's being marketed as advantageous for all people, all the time.

But although Fasting is healthy and safe for most people, some groups should steer clear. These groups comprise:

• children
• underweight people

• pregnant and nursing women

More food needs to be consumed by the above classes, not less. Any possible fasting benefits are outweighed by the possibility of nutrient deficiency.

Those with high blood sugar should proceed with caution as well. Although fasting for this population can be therapeutic, medical care is necessary in order to avoid the occurrence of dangerously low blood sugar (hypoglycemia).

Fasting Saps Your Energy

Food is fuel. Won't your energy levels plummet without it?

Ultimately, yes. But when you fast intermittently, your cells tap into an alternative energy source: body fat. And there are lots of that to go around.

That is right. Even a lean person has impressive fat reserves to meet energy needs when fasting (e.g., 150 pounds with 10 per cent body fat). If you do the math, 15 pounds of fat corresponds to more than 60,000 energy calories!

In reality, many individuals report better energy when they exercise in a fasting state. It makes sense, given that blood is redirected away from muscles and towards digestive organs after a large meal.

You Can't Focus While Fasting.

Think back to when you were ravenously hungry for the last time. Perhaps it wasn't your most Zen moment.

But if you follow a daily practice of intermittent Fasting, this "going to hangry" state should not be encountered. Your hunger hormones stabilize as your cells switch to using body fat for energy.

Burning body fat also produces ketones, tiny molecules that provide clean, effective energy to fuel your brain. It has been shown that promoting a state of ketosis enhances attention, concentration, and focus in older adults.

It's incredible what you can do for your body, brain, and health with this easy and versatile eating method.

Once you get beyond misinformed intermittent fasting misconceptions, you'll understand that many individuals end up achieving more while fasting. Many misconceptions concerning intermittent Fasting and the frequency of meals are perpetuated.

However, many of these rumours are not real.

For instance, eating smaller, more regular meals doesn't boost your metabolism or help you lose weight. Moreover, intermittent Fasting is far from unhealthy and could offer considerable benefits.

It's essential to consult sources or do a little research before jumping to conclusions about your metabolism and overall health.

Chapter 4: PROS and CONS of IF

There is a lot of preliminary fasting research pointing to some positive effects, but it needs much more research to back up the arguments.

One big advantage of Fasting is that it helps facilitate autophagy — a mechanism in which the cells eliminate damaged components effectively from the garbage. Increased autophagy will potentially regenerate the immune system and improve protection from stress for your cell.

Some evidence indicates that Fasting can also reduce blood pressure and make the body more insulin sensitive; being more insulin-sensitive means that you can be more effectively store energy from food and get less hungry between meals.

Now to the main reason, people are trying to fast — to lose weight. Although one study found that both fasting and caloric restriction (eating less all day long) resulted in the same weight loss outcomes, weight loss is a highly individual path. If you have struggled to find a way to eat that's helping you be your best self, you may want to try fasting.

Not surprisingly, the use of weight-loss Fasting has a long history. It makes sense that you are extremely likely to lose weight if you don't eat, which makes it even more shocking how many people are afraid of skipping even a single meal, let alone fasting for a day or more.

Some people are afraid that Fasting (not eating) will inevitably lead to a 'starvation state' and potentially make you fat. That's kind of like saying that you dry your hair by splashing water on your eyes. It is a mistruth that has been used to instil terror.

There are countless stories of people' ruining' their metabolism. Naturally, food producers have enthusiastically 'trained' medical professionals on the risks of skipping meals and on the health of consuming sugar. When you miss meals, nobody makes money.

Intermittent Fasting does not reflect a diet. Intermittent Fasting can bring health benefits, including weight loss, but it is not suitable for everyone.

Intermittent Fasting requires alternating between mealtimes and fasting periods. At first, people can find it difficult to eat each day within a short period or switch between eating days and not eating days.

Intermittent Fasting is a common approach that people use to simplify their lives, lose weight and improve overall health and wellbeing, including reducing the effects of ageing. It is a common choice of lifestyle that has potential benefits in terms of weight loss, body composition, disease prevention, and wellness.

Currently, chances are you have done several sporadic fasts before. Many people do this unconsciously, missing meals in the morning or in the evening.

An alternative would be to fast whenever it suits you. Occasionally missing meals when you don't feel hungry or have no time to prepare will work for some people.

It doesn't matter what kind of short you want at the end of the day. What's most important is discovering a strategy that works best for you and your lifestyle.

Most significantly, Intermittent Fasting is one of the easiest ways we must take off bad weight while retaining a healthy weight because it requires little change in behaviour.

Identify Personal Goals

An individual who begins intermittent Fasting usually has one target in mind. It can be about losing weight, improving physical health or improving metabolic health. The aim of an individual is to help them decide the most suitable form of Fasting and figure out how much calories and nutrients they need to eat.

Dieting is not fun; everyone can agree on that, but heading into the summer months means looking in the mirror and making some hard decisions. Rather than starving yourself by not eating enough of this or that, why not try Intermittent Fasting. Fasting in twelve-hour intervals has been shown to have a positive effect on weight loss, which is much better than it sounds if you're sleeping in between the hours. And any other day, you get to eat whatever you want, and yet so much.

If you are up to lose weight or improve overall health, recognize your needs before any diet or exercise program gets underway. Remember your lifestyle, and accordingly, develop your diet plan and meal schedules. Instead of setting unattainable goals, remember to set low, achievable goals that you can easily accomplish and step forward. Not being able to reach goals would just annoy you, so take it step by step.

Pick the Method

Consider how you want to accomplish your routine and short- or long-term goals once you have worked out your goals and caloric needs. Understand the basics of each form of intermittent fasting program and select the one you think would work for you. Usually, you would stick with each approach for at least a month or longer before trying another one to see whether it works for you or not.

Beyond that, remember to start slow — you want to become a better version of yourself, not fall ill after drastic diet plans!

An individual should choose the plan that fits their interests and that they feel they will stick to. Including:

• Eat Avoid Eat

• Diet Warrior

• Leangains 16:8

• Approaches 5:2

• Alternative fasts for the day

An individual will usually stick to a month or longer with one fasting method to see if it works for them before attempting another method. Those with a medical condition will talk with their healthcare provider before any fasting process starts.

An individual should note when deciding on a form that they don't need to consume a certain type or amount or type of food or avoid food altogether. An individual can eat whatever they want. However, it is a good idea to adopt a balanced, high-fibre, vegetable-rich diet during the eating periods to attain health and weight loss goals.

Binging on unhealthy foods over overeating days will hamper progress in health. Drinking loads of water or other non-calorie beverages is also extremely necessary during fast days.

Figure out Caloric Needs

Your body finds ways of extending your life when you're hungry. You want to gain weight; on the other hand, you need to be eating more calories than you are burning. To find out the calories and nutrients you are eating and what changes you need to make – there are many resources for the same. You should also receive advice from a dietitian.

The good news is that intermittent Fasting stimulates many of the same lifeextending pathways as calorie restriction. In other words, without the hassle of starving, you get the rewards of a longer life.

Intermittent Fasting is a term for meal timing schedules that includes voluntary Fasting or decreased calorie consumption over a given time and non-fasting. The regulated cycling between Fasting and eating is often called intermittent energy restriction and is a common form of weight loss. When fasting, there are no dietary limits, but that doesn't mean calories don't count.

Many people who do 5:2 intermittent Fasting consume between 500-600 calories two days a week and eat the other five days normally. When one of your goals is weight loss, this will help 0.5 – 1 pound weight loss per week, depending on your caloric needs. When you do 5:2 Fasting, making sure you eat high fibre meals and enough protein on non-fasting days is very necessary.

People who are trying to lose weight need to build their own calorie deficit — that means they consume fewer calories than they use—those who want to gain weight need to be eating more calories than they are carrying.

A lot of resources are available to help a person figure out their caloric needs and decide how many calories they need to eat every day to either gain or lose weight. An individual may also discuss how many calories they need with their health care provider or dietitian for guidance.

Typically, when people are strong, the only items they drink during the fasting time are plain black coffee, tea and water — for electrolytes, you can even add a dash of salt in the water. Many people assume, however, that eating something under 50 calories can keep you in a fasted state, so you can add a splash of heavy cream or oil into your coffee to help you tide over.

Intermittent Fasting helps to reduce calories and weight loss.

The primary reason prolonged weight loss fasting works is that it allows you to eat fewer calories.

The various procedures all include skipping meals during the fasting periods. If you compensate by drinking a lot more during the times of feeding, you would be consuming fewer calories.

Intermittent Fasting may result in weight loss, according to a recent 2014 review report. For this study, intermittent Fasting was observed over a span of 3-24 weeks to reduce body weight by 3-8 per cent. Participants lose around 0.55 pounds (0.25 kg) a week with intermittent Fasting while analyzing the rate of weight loss, but 1.65 pounds (0.75 kg) per week with alternate-day Fasting. People have lost 4-7% of their waist circumference, meaning they lost their belly fat.

Such findings are very promising and demonstrate that intermittent fasting can be effective in helping with weight loss.

All the advantages of intermittent fasting go well beyond just losing weight. It also has several metabolic health benefits and can even help to avoid chronic disease and extend lifespan.

While calorie counting is usually not needed when practising intermittent fasting, weight loss is often facilitated by a reduction in calorie intake overall.

Studies comparing intermittent Fasting and constant calorie restriction indicate little difference in weight loss when calories fit between classes.

Figure out A Meal Plan

An individual who is interested in losing or gaining weight may find it helpful to schedule what they will eat during the day or week.

Meal preparations should not be too restrictive. This takes calorie intake into account and integrates sufficient nutrients into the diet.

Meal preparation provides many benefits, such as having a person adhere to their calorie count and ensuring that they have the requisite food on hand to prepare recipes, fast meals and snack.

Make the Calories Count

Not all calories are the same. While these fasting methods do not set restrictions on how many calories a person should consume when fasting, consideration of the nutritional value of the food is essential.

An individual should generally strive to eat nutrient-dense foods or foods with a high number of nutrients per calorie. While a person does not have to give up junk food entirely, they still need to practice moderation and concentrate on more nutritious choices to reap the most benefits.

Know hunger moves like a stream. Don't worry about your hunger being intolerable; you'll be okay if you ignore it and turn your attention into work or other activities. On the second day, when you fast for an extended period, hunger often increases, but it begins to gradually recede. You should expect a total loss of hunger sensation by the third or fourth day while your body stays motivated by stored body fat!

Most importantly, remember to stay hydrated as often. The only thirst is what you perceive as hunger. I prefer natural sweeteners and flavour enhancers such as spices and herbs over sugar or just take more calories.

Keys for Success

For those of you interested in Fasting, remember that some key factors help you to make the best of your fasts. These are much important to remember; some of those keys for success are:

Electrical Energy

Electrical Energy is one aspect that is often overlooked, and it's very important to bring this to your attention at this time.

The first thing we think of when people talk about energy is our caloric needs. How much carbohydrates, fat, and protein we need to eat to get the strength we need to live every day. The one extremely critical item never mentioned, but most importantly, is Electrical Energy.

Electrical energy gives life to every cell in our body, and for us to be alive, it is essential. The way to maximize your electric power is to eat as many raw vegetables and fruit as possible.

Fat

Fat is one source of energy. Next, your body will burn carbohydrates, so it will start consuming your fat supply when that's exhausting.

You will find fat in foods like nuts, seeds, meat, oil, very yummy avocado, fish and some butter.

There are two different kinds of fat, the healthy type called monounsaturated fatty acids found in oils, the polyunsaturated fatty acids found in plant-based foods, and the Omega-3 found in fatty fish such as salmon.
Then there are the harmful ones found in animal products called saturated fats and Trans fats that come from refined oils.

Carbohydrates

Carbs are in your dairy, vegetables, fruits and cereals almost everywhere!

The good form called Complex Carbohydrates is found in beans, vegetables and whole grains. But these too are converted into glucose when we eat too much, which is contained in body fat.

Then there are the poor ones in candy, white sugar, white flour, white rice, to name a few, called Simple Carbohydrates. Your body uses this first for a source of energy, and if it can't use all of it, it will store it and make you fat, as described above.

Protein

Protein makes up your body, your hair, your nails and your skin.

Protein can be contained in poultry, eggs, fish, nutmeg, nuts, wheat, beans, soy, broccoli, etc. Without protein, we cannot live.

How to Count Macros

When you look at nutritional statistics, it says calories per serving, how big the serving is, with everything expressed in grams of fat, carbohydrates and protein.

How many calories a gram has to offer?

Proteins account for four calories per gram.

Carbs contain four calories per gram.

Fats are nine calories a gram.
Why counting macros is more critical than simply calorie counting.

Although without the other, Macronutrients and Calories cannot exist. Macronutrients form calories and go hand in hand.

It's not a good idea to only count calories, consume whatever you like, as long as the number of calories you're allowed to eat doesn't surpass that.

You have to pay attention to the food's nutrient content, and this is where macros counting come in.

Calorie counting can leave you hungry and sometimes lead to over-eating.

Not always are calorie-rich foods full.

Knowing what your perfect ratios of macros are will lead you to consume the right foods.

200 Broccoli calories have a higher caloric value than a 200-calorie piece of cake.

In choosing nutrient-rich foods, you need to make the most of what you put into your mouth and into your body.

Macro Ratio

You need to find out first what your Total Daily Expenditure on Energy (TDEE) is to maintain your weight. You will go to various online TDEE calculators.

Your Macros ratio is something of an individual nature. It depends on what you want. By now, you have met your target weight, and you're going to decide if you want to keep your weight or tone up and gain muscle.

Macros to maintain weight ratio
- Fat – 25% to 40%
- Protein – 25% to 40%
- Carbohydrates – 35% to 55%

Based on this, you will choose your ratios to be up to 100%. If you have or have diabetes, a tendency to become diabetic, then hold down to a minimum the percentage of Carb. Perhaps even smaller, 25 per cent and your fat ratio will increase.

Macros to gain muscular ratio

- Fat – 20% Fat
- Proteins – 35%
- Carbohydrates – 45%

High protein and high Carb ratio, as you are going to work out muscle building.

The context for measuring weight maintenance macros

Say you're 50 years of age, 5'5" tall, weigh 155 pounds, and you're engaged in moderation.

Your TDEE is calorie 1721. This is the number of calories you will need to hold your weight.

For weight maintenance, the required macronutrient ratio is:

- 25 – 40 % of fat
- 35 – 55 % of carbohydrates
- 25 – 40 % of protein

Carbohydrates have a bad rap, so keep it at least 35%.

Fat is delicious so let's set this at 35%.
30% protein because you are moderately active.

If you get 1721 calories required:

35 percent Fat are: 1721 x 0,35 = 602 calories per day.

30 percent Protein are: 1721 x 0,30 = 516 calories per day.

35 percent Carbs are: 1721 x 0,35 = 602 calories per day.

Breaking it to grams

Fat comes with nine calories per gram. 602: 9 = 67 grams of fat average

Protein comes with four calories per gram. 516: 4 = 129 grams per day of protein

Carbs contain four calories per gram. 602: 4 = 151 grams of carbs a day

Here are the most relevant principles of Intermittent Fasting:

When to Eat

Divide your day into two blocks of time, one to eat and the other too fast. You don't have to be obsessed with calories like intermittent Fasting lunatic. It is not a material diet, as explained above. It's a diet that is timing meals.

As you hit the later stages of a short-term fast, normally 12-16 hours a day, your body starts increasing the secretion of natural growth hormones and other hormones that control appetite and body fats. It also affects the sugar in the blood and how the body replaces its cells.

So, when is it that you should eat? First of all, you have to consider how long you want to keep your fast every day. For first-timers, 12 hours is a bare minimum and ideal, and 20 hours is considered extreme.
All you need to do then is separate your day into time frames for "eating" and non-eating. So, if you're fasting for twelve hours and start eating at 8 a.m., you have all your daily calories to consume before 8 p.m.

Once you enter the non-eating time frame, you will not be allowed to consume any more calories until the morning afterwards.

What to Eat

Intermittent Fasting doesn't need to work with particular foods or diets. Once you have decided how long each day you want to fast, it is time to decide which content you want to consume. Unlike other diets, there is no set rule with respect to what sort of food you consume.

This makes intermittent Fasting highly versatile and enables it to be paired with other food philosophies such as Low Carb, vegetarian, and simply healthy eating.

Since your hormones, blood sugar, and other weight loss factors do all the heavy lifting for you, it's not important to join a big calorie deficit.

Even on intermittent Fasting, sadly, you can't live in a calorie surplus and lose weight. A minimum 200 calorie deficit is more than enough to effectively lose weight.

Many dieters lost weight and gained leaner while using intermittent Fasting without limiting calories. In other words, they didn't change what they ate every day; they only followed the time periods for eating and not eating without major changes to the average calorie count. The bigger your calorie deficit, the greater the weight loss you can expect. Here are some essential food items you can eat.

Medical advantages of Fasting

At the point when you don't eat any nourishment for a set timeframe every day, you do your body and your mind a mess of good. It bodes well from a developmental angle. For the vast majority of history, individuals weren't eating three nourishing meals daily, in addition to consuming snacks. Rather, people developed in circumstances where there wasn't a lot of nourishment, and they figured out how to flourish when fasting. These days, we don't need to chase for nourishment (in spite of the fact that chasing for your very own meat is anything but an ill-conceived notion!). Or maybe, we go through a large portion of our days before PCs, and we eat at whatever point we need — despite the fact that our bodies aren't adjusted to this conduct.

Changing to a discontinuous fasting diet grows your points of confinement and lifts your exhibition in various ways.

The advantages of irregular Fasting:

- Boosts weight reduction
- Increases vitality
- Promotes cell fix and autophagy (when your body expends faulty tissue so as to create new parts)
- Reduces insulin opposition and ensures against type 2 diabetes
- Lowers terrible cholesterol
- Promotes life span
- Protects against neurodegenerative maladies, for example, Alzheimer's and Parkinson's
- Improves memory and lifts mind work
- Makes cells stronger

Numerous studies have been done on irregular Fasting in creatures and people. These examinations have demonstrated that it can have groundbreaking benefits for weight control and the wellbeing of your body and mind. It might even assist you with living longer.

Here are the primary medical advantages of discontinuous Fasting:

- Weight misfortune: As referenced above, discontinuous Fasting can assist you in getting more fit and lose fat without having to deliberately limit calories (1, 13Trusted Source).
- Insulin obstruction: Intermittent Fasting can diminish insulin opposition, bringing down glucose by 3–6% and fasting insulin levels by 20–31%, which ought to ensure against type 2 diabetes. • Inflammation: Some examinations show decreases in markers of irritation, a key driver of numerous incessant infections. • Heart

wellbeing: Intermittent Fasting may decrease "awful" LDL cholesterol, blood triglycerides, incendiary markers, glucose, and insulin obstruction — all hazard factors for coronary illness. • Cancer: Animal investigations propose that irregular Fasting may anticipate malignant growth.

- Brain wellbeing: Intermittent Fasting expands the cerebrum hormone BDNF and may help the development of new nerve cells. It might likewise ensure against Alzheimer's sickness.
- Anti-maturing: Intermittent Fasting can expand life expectancy in rodents. Studies demonstrated that fasted rodents lived 36–83% longer.

Remember that exploration is still in its beginning periods. A large number of the investigations were little, present moment, or led in creatures. Numerous inquiries presently can't seem to be replicated in more relevant human examinations. Rundown Intermittent Fasting can have numerous advantages for your body and cerebrum. It can cause weight reduction and may diminish your danger of type 2 diabetes, coronary illness, and disease. It might likewise assist you with living longer.

Chapter 5: Intermittent fasting for a woman over 50

Intermittent Fasting is beneficial for most people who eat during their daytime hours. Prolonged Fasting differs from the usual eating style. If someone consumes three meals per day, including treats, and they don't work out, they operate on certain calories and don't burn their fat reserves at any time. Intermittent Fasting allows our bodies to burn the reserved fat storage healthily; nine older women in ten have a form of chronic illness, and nearly eight in ten have more than one chronic disease. So, odds are, eventually, a person will get more. But to live a healthy life, there are measures one should take, and fasting intermittently is one of them.

Many of these chronic illnesses start from being overweight at an older age. The most important aspect of intermittent Fasting is its weight loss assistance. Another research found that intermittent Fasting induces less muscle loss than the more traditional daily restriction of calories. Bear in mind, though, that the primary explanation for its effectiveness is that intermittent Fasting allows you to intake fewer calories overall. During your meal times, if you indulge and consume large quantities, you will not lose much weight at all.

Why Start Intermittent Fasting After 50?

Here, excess weight in women can cause several diseases, and intermittent Fasting can help counteract them. Furthermore, intermittent fasting can help you control these aspects of living if you are over 50.

• Hypertension

Blood vessels become less elastic when a person grows older. This puts a strain on the mechanism that holds the body's blood. It may indicate why 2 in 3 women over the age of 50 have elevated blood pressure.

• Diabetes

At least one in 10 women has diabetes. When you grow older, the odds of having the disease increase up. Heart failure, renal disease, blindness, and other complications may arise from diabetes due to excess weight.

•Cardiac Condition

A significant source of heart attack is plaque formation in the arteries due to unhealthy eating. It begins in youth, and as one matures, it becomes worse. A large percentage of men and 5.6 per cent of women have suffered from heart failure in the 40-58 age range in the U.S. Fasting and eating healthy is a good option to control any cardiovascular diseases

• Obesity

It might be dangerous for the health if one weighs too much for their height; it's not about getting a few extra pounds. More than 20 obesity chronic illnesses are correlated with stroke, asthma, arthritis, cancer, coronary failure, and high blood pressure. At least 30% of the older population is obese.

•Arthritis

This condition of the joints was once directly attributed by physicians to the excessive wear and tear of time, and it sure is a cause. Yet biology and lifestyle are likely to have still much to do with it. A lack of physical exercise, diabetes, and becoming overweight may play a role in past joint accidents, too.

•Osteoporosis

With old age, bones become weak, especially in women, which may lead to fractures. It impacts nearly 53.9 million Americans over 50 years of age. A few factors that will help are-a balanced diet high in vitamin D and

Calcium, losing excess weight by fasting, and daily weight-bearing activity, such as walking, jogging, and climbing stairs.

•Tumor & Cancers

The greatest risk factor for old age is cancer. The disorder also impacts young adults, but between 46 and 54 years of age, you risk getting it more than doubles. You can't influence a person's age or genes, but you choose stuff like smoking or living an unhealthy lifestyle. With much of the study focusing on the beneficial impact, fasting has on cancer, fasting over varying periods of time has often helped older women decrease their risk of severe diseases. The study reported that Fasting appears to suppress some cancer-causing pathways and can even delay tumour development.

• Menopause

The classic indicators of menopause are hot flashes, insomnia, night sweats, mood swings, vaginal dryness, burning, and itching. Heart failure and osteoporosis appear to escalate throughout the years of menopause. Often people start prolonged Fasting to combat both the long-term and short-term symptoms of menopause. For several post-menopausal women, Belly fat, not just for appearance but also for health, is a major concern. The decrease in belly fat resulting from intermittent Fasting helps women minimize their likelihood of metabolic syndrome, a series of health conditions that enhance the risk of heart disease and diabetes for a post-menopausal female.

Advantages of Intermittent Fasting for Women Over 50

The benefits of intermittent Fasting for women over 50 are limitless; some of them are mentioned here:

A decrease in insulin resistance-Fasting is one of the most successful strategies to return the insulin receptors to a normal sensitivity level. Understanding the role insulin plays is one of the biggest keys to learning about Fasting and truly understanding every diet. Concerning eating, insulin, the hormone that controls blood sugar, is formed in the pancreas and absorbed into the bloodstream. Insulin allows the body to retain energy as fat until released. Insulin creates fat because the more fat the body stores, the more insulin the body makes or vice versa. The cycles during which a person is not eating allow the body time to reduce insulin levels, mainly during intermittent Fasting, which changes the fat-storing mechanism. The mechanism goes in reverse, and the body loses weight as insulin levels decrease.

Autophagy is the incredible way the cells "eat themselves" to eliminate dead cells and recycle the younger parts. Autophagy is often the mechanism by which harmful pathogens, including viruses, bacteria, and other diseases, are killed. As the whole cell is recycled, another step in apoptosis, your chance of getting cancer rises without this process when defective cells tend to multiply.

Intermittent Fasting leads to Detoxification. Many of us have been subjected to contaminants from food and our climate in our lifetime. Many of these contaminants are processed in our bodies in fat cells. One of the most powerful methods to eliminate contaminants from the body is fasting and eating healthy.

- The body's internal clock or Circadian Rhythm of the body controlsvirtually any mechanism in the body, and a chain of detrimental results will occur when it is disturbed. You adjust the circadian clock of the body while you take a rest from meals.

- A Healthy Gut is one of Fasting's most important aspects, as Fastingprovides a chance for the digestive tract and intestinal flora to reset. This is critical because the health of the body's digestive system regulates the immune system. There is even more proof that one's moods and emotional wellbeing are co-dependent on the gut microbiota. In recent studies of any area related to health and wellbeing, there has been a lot of hype on how one's gut flora might play an important part. The work of a more powerful immune system is important to a diverse microbiota, and it plays an important role in one's mental wellbeing. It also removes skin problems and reduces cancer danger. Although the foods you consume have an immense effect on your intestinal health, periodic Fasting in the digestive system can be another way to help grow the beneficial bacteria in the gut. Sugar and artificial goods disturb the equilibrium of your digestive tract between the beneficial and detrimental microbiota. Make sure to minimize packaged foods full of refined carbohydrates, sugars, and harmful fats to get the best outcome if you try Intermittent Fasting. Alternatively, switch to whole grains, plenty of organic vegetables and fruits, and good quality protein.

- Intermittent Fasting will work better by metabolic switching. Fastingcontributes to lower glucose levels in the bloodstream. The body utilizes fat as an energy source instead of sugar after converting the fat into ketones.

- Although it's not fasting, several physicians have recorded intermittentfasting advantages by permitting some easy-to-digest foods during the fasting window as fresh fruit. Modifications like this will also provide the essential rest for your metabolic and digestive system.

• Losing weight-It is expected that Fasting helps accelerate the loss of excess weight. It also decreases insulin levels such that the body no longer receives the message to store more calories as fat during the state of Fasting. Intermittent Fasting may contribute to a self-activating decrease in calorie consumption by letting you consume fewer meals. Besides, to promote weight reduction, prolonged Fasting affects hormone levels. It enhances noradrenaline or norepinephrine production, which is a fatburning hormone, lowering insulin and raising growth hormone levels. Intermittent Fasting can increase one's metabolic rate due to these changes in hormones. By encouraging one to eat less and activating ketones' production, intermittent Fasting induces weight loss by adjusting all calorie calculation factors. In contrast to other weight loss trials, a study showed that this eating method would cause 3-8 per cent weight loss in just weeks, which is a substantial percentage. People have lost 4 to 7 per cent of their waist circumference; as per the same report, it helps women dealing with menopause and unhealthy stomach fat that builds up over their organs and induces illness.

Other than insulin, during intermittent Fasting are two important hormones, leptin and ghrelin. Ghrelin is the hormone of starvation that tells the body when it's hungry. Research shows that ghrelin can be reduced by Intermittent Fasting. There is also some evidence suggesting a rise in the leptin hormone, the hormone of satiety. That tells the body when it's full, and there's no more urge to eat.

• People would be fuller quicker and hungry less frequently with lessghrelin and more leptin, which may lead to fewer calories eaten and, as a result, weight loss.

Other benefits of intermittent Fasting in women over 50 are stated hereunder: • Alzheimer's

Alzheimer's disorder in women over 50 and other neurodegenerative diseases may be severe. There are many lifestyle options that scientists claim, including extended Fasting, may help avoid Alzheimer's. Recent research released says prolonged Fasting preserves the polarization of aquaporin-4 in the brain. It can help defend against Alzheimer's. Aquaporin-4 plays a key function in eliminating amyloid-β, a peptide thought to contribute to Alzheimer's. Intermittent Fasting may be one of the best approaches to lower the risk of Alzheimer's, getting a brain boost alongside a well-balanced diet and daily exercise.

•Depression & Intermittent Fasting

Personal wellbeing factors are taken into account in the evaluation research. Several findings show that women who follow distinct fasting strategies reported changes in their moods for better self-esteem, reducing depression and anxiety.

• IF Increases Joint & Muscle Health

According to research, Fasting increases muscle and joint protection because low back pain and arthritic symptoms were not as prominent.

•Inflammation Reduction

According to research, many women over 50 during intermittent Fasting reported that they had achieved a decline in oxidative stress and inflammation, which is extremely significant, considering the vast number of women who had breast cancer family history. There is also not an increase in ghrelin, the hormone of hunger, which is beneficial.

•Maintaining Metabolism

A decrease in the resting rate of metabolic or 'metabolism' is one issue that can occur with weight loss. It makes it difficult to lose weight as this happens; the body doesn't burn many calories. Still, intermittent Fasting helps the metabolism rate increase so that women over 50 easily lose excess weight with Fasting.

IF also improves LDL cholesterol, total cholesterol and triglycerides, and blood pressure for the better. The same advantages are experienced by the women doing 5:2 Fasting or any other way of intermittent Fasting. With daily alternating Fasting, both women and men can experience a substantial drop in insulin, increased ketones, and unsaturated fatty acids, meaning that women would benefit as much as men.

As a woman over 50, you can maximize intermittent fasting advantages by following these few points:

Sugar and processed grains should be avoided. Eat apples, whole grains, vegetables, beans, lean proteins, lentils, and good fats (a good, Mediterranean-style diet based on plants).

Between meals, let the body burn fat. Don't snack on unhealthy foods. During your day, be productive. Develop your lean muscles.

• Consider a more effective form of Intermittent Fasting. Restrict the day's hours to consume calories, and make it early in the day for a better effect.

Avoid getting sweets or consuming all the time at night.
Besides, certain senior women may need to consume food daily due to their metabolic conditions or prescription guidelines; under any scenario, a person should address their dietary patterns with care practitioners before making any adjustments.

Potential Risks of Intermittent Fasting for Women Over 50

Certainly, prolonged Fasting might not be for everyone. If you are undernourished or have a record of eating disorders, you must not start intermittent fast without first speaking with a health provider. There is some proof that intermittent Fasting for some women might not be as effective for men. For instance, one research found that it increased insulin sensitivity in males than females. Still, in certain women that blood sugar regulation worsens; it may be because of some women's underlying condition.

You should contact a doctor before attempting intermittent Fasting if you have a medical problem. It is especially relevant for you if you

• Take medications.

• Have diabetes

• Have problems with blood sugar regulation.

• Are underweight.

• Have a history of eating disorders

• Have a history of amenorrhea

• Have low blood pressure.

Although intermittent Fasting shows potential, we don't have clear proof of the long-term impact of how often older adults might be influenced by Fasting. Human experiments have mainly focused on categories including middle-aged and young people for a brief amount of time. Yet, we do know that, in certain situations, intermittent Fasting might be dangerous. As far as low body weight is concerned, it is worrisome that a person would lose so much weight, impacting their bones, energy level, and overall immune system.

According to doctors, People who need their medication to survive with food to prevent discomfort or stomach irritation cannot do well with Intermittent Fasting. People who take cardiac or blood pressure drugs may also be more likely to develop harmful sodium and potassium imbalances as they try to fast.

If you have diabetes and require food after some hours or taking medicine that influences your blood sugar, intermittent Fasting can even be dangerous.

If intermittent Fasting is important for wellbeing, causing you hunger, pangs will interrupt sleep. It could even render you less conscious or aware. Intermittent Fasting will contribute to reducing alertness since the body does not eat sufficient calories to provide enough nutrition during a fasting window. Fasting can also contribute to tiredness, problems focusing, or dizziness.

If you leave the fast too early, the diet does not entail guilt or self-shaming —a potential sign of disordered behaviour, maybe some form of fear or embarrassment surrounding your fast.

While intermittent fasting is a very beneficial solution for women over 50, you can also rethink intermittent Fasting if you notice these symptoms and signs:

• It could be linked to Fasting if someone experiences hair loss.

• In the starting stages of intermittent Fasting, thirst, exhaustion, and fatigueare very common.

- During the feeding time, overeating or not eating nutritious foods leads toextreme hunger.

- Heartburn or reflux owing to heavy eating.

A hint that Intermittent Fasting may not be safe for you is the feelings of fear, sadness, or anti-social emotions.

While intermittent Fasting is not inherently harmful, individuals with an eating condition or family or a personal background must stay clear of the diet. For those extremely active, intermittent Fasting is also not suitable because they need more energy.

Food gives our body movement energy, so exercising while Fasting will impact efficiency and contribute to an unsafe energy deficiency. Focus on healthy, nutrient-packed options, such as fruits, veggies, lean meats, legumes, and whole grains, while some experts often combine IF with keto or low-carb or keto diet types. Assume that you will cope with lower stamina, cravings, and bloating before the body changes for the first several weeks.

Chapter 6: Types of IF

16/8 Method

This is just about the most popular fasting methods since it's so schedule based, meaning there are no surprises. This will give you the freedom to control when you eat based on the everyday life of yours. The sixteen is the number of hours you're likely to be fasting, which may also be lowered to twelve or perhaps fourteen hours if that fits into your life better. Then your eating period is going to be between eight and ten hours every day. This might seem daunting, but it just means that you are skipping an entire meal. Many people choose to begin their fast around 7 or 8 p.m. and then do not eat until 11 or noon the next day, which means they fast for the recommended 16 hours. Of course, it isn't as bad as it sounds since they are sleeping during this time, so what it comes down to is eating dinner and then not eating the next day again around lunch, so you are just skipping breakfast.

You will be doing it every day, so finding the hours that work for you are important. If you work the third shift, then switching your eating period around to fit into your schedule is important. If you find yourself being run down and sluggish, tweak your fasting hours until you find a healthy balance. Granted, there will be some adjustment because chances are, your body is not accustomed to skipping entire meals. However, this should go away after a couple of weeks, and if it doesn't, then try starting your fasting period earlier in the day, allowing you to eat earlier the next, or alter it however you need to feel healthy and happy.

Lean-Gains Method (14:10)

The lean-gains method has several different incarnations on the web, but its fame comes from the fact that it helps shed fat while building it into muscle almost immediately. Through the lean-gains method, you'll find yourself able to shift all that fat to be muscle through a rigorous practice of fasting, eating right, and exercising.

Through this method, you fast anywhere from 14 to 16 hours and spend the remaining 10 or 8 hours each day engaged in eating and exercise. As opposed to the crescendo, this method features daily fasting and eating, rather than alternated days of eating versus not. Therefore, you don't have to be quite cautious about extending the physical effort to exercise on the days you are fasting because those days when you're fasting are every day!

For the lean-gaining method, start fasting only for 14 hours and work it up to 16 if you feel comfortable with it, but never forget to drink enough water and be careful about spending too much energy on exercise! Remember that you want to grow in health and potential through intermittent fasting. You'll certainly not want to lose any of that growth by forcing the process along.

20:4 Method

Stepping things up a notch from the 14:10 and 16:8 methods, the 20:4 method is a tough one to master, for it is rather unforgiving. People talk about this method of intermittent fasting as intense and highly restrictive. Still, they also say that the effects of living this method are almost unparalleled with all other tactics.

For the 20:4 method, you'll fast for 20 hours each day and squeeze all your meals, all your eating, and all your snacking into 4 hours. People who attempt 20:4 normally have two smaller meals or just one large meal and a few snacks during their 4-hour window to eat, and it is up to the individual which four hours of the day they devote to eating.

The trick for this method is to make sure you're not overeating or bingeing during those 4-hour windows to eat. It is all-too-easy to get hungry during the 20-hour fast and have that feeling then propel you into intense and unrealistic hunger or meal sizes after the fast period is over. Be careful if you try this method. If you're new to intermittent fasting, work your way up to this one gradually, and if you're working your way up already, only make the shift to 20:4 when you know you're ready. It would surely disappoint if all your progress with intermittent fasting got hijacked by one poorly thought-out goal with the 20:4 method.

Meal Skipping

Meal skipping is an extremely flexible form of intermittent fasting that can provide all of the benefits of intermittent fasting but with less strict scheduling. If you are not someone who has a typical schedule or feels like a more strict variation of the intermittent fasting diet will serve you, meal skipping is a viable alternative.

Many people who choose to use meal skipping find it a great way to listen to their bodies and follow their basic instincts. If they are not hungry, they simply don't eat that meal. Instead, they wait for the next one. Meal skipping can also help people who have time constraints and who may not always be able to get in a certain meal of the day.

It is important to realize that with meal skipping, you may not always be maintaining a 10-16-hour window of fasting. As a result, you may not get every benefit that comes from other fasting diets. However, this may be a great solution for people who want an intermittent fasting diet that feels more natural. It may also be a great idea for those looking to begin listening to their bodies more so that they can adjust to a more intense variation of the diet with greater ease. It can be a great transitional diet for you if you are not ready to jump into one of the other fasting diets just yet.

Warrior Diet Fasting

The most extreme form of intermittent fasting is known as the Warrior Diet. This intermittent fasting cycle follows a 20-hour fasting window with a short 4-hour eating window. During that eating window, individuals are supposed to only consume raw fruits and vegetables. They can also eat one large meal. Typically, the eating window occurs at night time, so people can snack throughout the evening, have a large meal, and then resume fasting.

Because of the length of fasting taking place during the Warrior Diet, people should also consume a fairly hearty level of healthy fats. Doing so will give the body something to consume during the fast to produce energy with. A small number of carbohydrates can also be incorporated to support energy levels too.

People who eat the Warrior Diet tend to believe that humans are natural nocturnal eaters and that we are not meant to eat throughout the day. The belief is that eating this way follows our natural circadian rhythms, allowing our body to work optimally.

The only people who should consider doing the Warrior Diet are those who have already had success with other forms of intermittent fasting and who are used to it. Attempting to jump straight into the Warrior Diet can have serious repercussions for anyone who is not used to intermittent fasting. Even still, those who are used to it may find this particular style too extreme for them to maintain.

Eat-Stop-Eat (24 Hour) Method

This method of fasting is incredibly similar to the crescendo method. The only discernable difference is that there's no anticipation of increasing into a more intense fasting pattern with time. For the eat-stop-eat method, you decide which days you want to take off from eating, and then you run with it until you've lost that weight, and then you keep running with the lifestyle for good because you won't be able to imagine life without it.

The eat-stop-eat method involves one to two days a week being 100% oriented towards fasting, with the other five to six days concerning "business as normal." The one or two days spent fasting are then full 24hour days spent without eating anything at all. These days, of course, water and coffee are still fine to drink, but no food items can be consumed whatsoever. Exercise is also frowned upon on those fasting days but see what your body can handle before you decide how that should all work out.

Some people might start thinking they're using the crescendo method but end up sticking with eat-stop-eat.

Alternate-Day Method

The alternate-day method is admittedly a little confusing, but the reason it could be so confusing could come, in part, from how much wiggle room it provides for the practitioner. This method is great for people who don't have a consistent schedule or any sense of one, and it is incredibly forgiving for those who don't quite have everything together for themselves yet.

When it comes down to it, alternate-day intermittent fasting is really up to you. You should try to fast every other day, but it doesn't have to be that precise. Similarly, with the crescendo method, as long as you fast two to three days a week, with a break day or two in between each fasting day, you're set! Then, you'll want to eat normally for three or four days out of each week, and when you encounter a fasting day, you don't even need to completely fast!

Alternate-day fasting is a solid place to start from, especially if you work a varying schedule or still have yet to get used to a consistent one. If you want to make things more intense from this starting point, the alternate-day method can easily become the eat-stop-eat method, the crescendo method, or the 5:2 method. Essentially, this method is a great place to begin.

12:12 Method

As another of the more natural ways of intermittent fasting, the 12:12 approach is well-suited to beginning practitioners. Many people live out the 12:12 method without any forethought simply because of their sleeping and eating schedule, but turning 12:12 into a conscious practise can have just as many positive effects on your life as the more drastic 20:4 method claims.

According to a study conducted in the University of Alabama, For this method, in particular, you fast for 12 hours and then enter a 12-hour eating window. It's not difficult whatsoever to get three small meals and several snacks, or two big meals and a snack into your day with this method. At 12:12, the standard meal timing works just fine.

Ultimately, this method is a great one to start from, for a lot of variation can be built into this scheduling when you're ready to make things more interesting. Effortlessly and without much effort, 12:12 can become 14:10 or even 16:8, and in seemingly no time, you can find yourself trying alternate-day or crescendo methods, too. Start with what's normal for you, and this method might be exactly that!

Chapter 7: Tips & tricks

Stay hydrated. Drink plenty of beverages that are free of calories, such as water, herbal teas, during the day—avoiding a fascination with food. You must plan your fasting day around activities you enjoy, so you will not be thinking about food or obsessing over what you will eat next.

Resting & Relaxation. On fasting days, you should not do strenuous exercises; however, light physical activities such as yoga and walking around the house can be helpful.

Make each calorie count. Now that you have chosen a plan for intermittent fasting, it is necessary to eat every calorie as nutrient-rich as possible. Select foods that are rich in fibre, good lean protein, and healthy fats. Nuts, Corn, lentils, poultry, pork, fish, and avocado are some examples.

You are consuming high-volume products. You must eat nutrient-packed high-volume foods, but for snacking, also look for low-calorie foods such as melons, grapes, vegetables with high water content, fruits or popcorn.

Improve the flavour without the calories. Generously season your meals with flavour-packed garlic, vegetables, sauces, or spices and fresh herbs. These spices are low-calorie but rich in flavour and will help in feeling less hungry. Select foods that are nutrient-dense during fasting time.

Consuming diets that are rich in fibre, vitamins, minerals, and other nutrients tend to maintain blood sugar levels stable and avoid nutritional deficiencies. A healthy diet can also lead to weight reduction and good well-being.

If you want to do the 16:8 intermittent fasting, here are the tips that people find useful:

- Drink herbal cinnamon tea throughout the fasting time because it reducesthe appetite

- Consume water periodically during the day

- Watch minimal television to decrease sensitivity to food pictures that maystimulate a feeling of hunger

- Work out only before or during the feeding window, since exercise willcontribute to hunger

- Try to eat thoughtful nutrition-packed food after breaking fast. Trymeditation to encourage hunger pangs to pass throughout the fasting time.

Speak to your doctor if you're thinking about attempting intermittent fasting, particularly if you already have health problems such as heart conditions and diabetes. Expert advises trying to take it easy with the diet. The time window for feeding is shortened steadily over many months.

Also, as the specialist has advised, continue the medication routine. It doesn't interrupt the fast to take drugs and take the medication with caloriefree beverages like black coffee and water.

• What if you require food with medicines?

You may try to modify the fast in that case. It has been shown that overweight individuals can always do a lot of good even by taking medication with small portions of food. Work out a prescription with your practitioner that would support your wellbeing without losing the benefits.

You would like to ease into whether you plan to attempt a fat fast or do intense intermittent fasting. If you are already consuming an unhealthy diet packed with quick snacks, fatty foods, and refined carbohydrates, you don't want to rush into these extreme fasts. One will find themselves in the bathroom for much of the day if you try to rush into fasting. Instead, by first performing a 16:8 fast on its own and keeping off the junk food, build your way up to doing these intense ways of intermittent fasting. Some literature speaks of doing a fat fast over a few days up to several weeks at a time.

• Your subconscious is the greatest barrier.

It's really easy to follow this plan. You simply should not eat until you wake up. Then you have lunch and dinner, and then you go on your day.

• Weight loss is simple.

If you consume less frequently, you will prefer to eat less in general. As a consequence, most people that pursue intermittent fasting wind-up losing weight. You might be preparing large meals, but in reality, consuming them regularly is tough. Keep monitoring what healthy foods make you feel better during fasting, and keep cycling them. Intermittent fasting helps, but before a person incorporates carb cycling and calorie cycling, some people did not lose weight. By consuming a lot on the days, you exercise and eat less on the days you do not exercise, you cycle calories.

• Prepare to get a lot of water to drink.

For you, the safest lifestyle is the one that fits you.

Pay Attention to These Things When Starting Intermittent Fasting Over 50

One might find themselves grappling with hunger pangs as of a fasting novice. Don't worry; once the body gets used to intermittent fasting, these are going to vanish.

Ensure that one drinks enough water, particularly throughout the fasting window, during the day. Water can help keep headaches at ease, which will encourage you to stay feeling full. Tea, black coffee, and low sodium bone broth are other drinks you can drink. Remember not to add milk or sugar to coffee and tea, or your fast won't do you any good.

Until you have achieved your fast, do not be pressured to overeat. Plan in advance: Load the plate with fresh, nutrient-packed foods full of highquality lean proteins, fibre, and good fats instead of bingeing on anything in view. After the fast is over, these healthy meals will hold you sated and less inclined to overeat.

Here are some frequently thought-out questions for people over 50.

During the fast, can one drink liquids?

Yes. It is good to have water, tea, black coffee, and other non-caloric drinks. Do not add the cream to coffee. There could be tiny quantities of milk or cream that are okay. They must be non-fattening. During a fast, coffee may be especially helpful, as it can curb hunger.

Is missing breakfast unhealthy?

No. The concern is that there are unsafe lifestyles for most traditional breakfast skippers. If you make sure that for the remainder of the day, you consume nutritious food, so fasting is healthy.

When fasting, should one take supplements?

Yes. Bear in mind, though, that certain supplements can function best when taken with meals, such as fat-soluble vitamins, so look out for that.

Can an individual exercise while fasting?

Yes, easy workouts are okay. But remember not to overexert yourself. For women over 50, simple yoga, brisk walking around the house, cleaning also count as work out. Yeah, easy workouts are okay.

Would fasting trigger muscle loss?

All forms of weight reduction can induce muscle loss, so lifting weights and maintaining your protein consumption is crucial. One research found that intermittent fasting induces less loss of muscle than a daily restriction of calories.

Can the Metabolism Slow down during Fasting?

No. Studies indicate that short-term fasting improves metabolism. Lengthier fasts of three or more days, therefore, can suppress and disrupt metabolism.

Chapter 8: Preparation to IF

In as much as intermittent fasting is famous for helping you lose weight, simplifying your life, and even improving your health in general, it's a timed approach to eating and not like being on a diet.

Therefore, intermittent fasting might not be proper for people with any medical condition, just as it is safe for well-nourished, healthy individuals. Consider these tips as a guide to aid you in starting your fast and starting it right.

What are your personal goals?

Clearly, you must have a goal – your reason for starting the fast, and this must be properly defined in your mind. Your reason for the fast will help you decide the right methods of fasting to employ so as to work on the nutrients and calories level required by your body.

Ease into it

Don't go about fasting for 14 days when you have never fasted before. Start off with 12 hours, and if it goes well, then you can take it up a notch, say 24 hours, then three days, and so on. Be realistic here. If you know that from your waking moment till when you retire to bed, food never leaves your mouth, start gradually, then grow into it as you experience progress.

Choose the method

As long as the goal has been clearly defined, the method of fasting becomes next. It is recommended that you try out a fasting method for a month or so before moving to the next. Since the methods of fasting are of four types, go for the one that best meets the demands of your health.

An individual should choose and stick with one of the following methods: eat-stop-eat, Warrior Diet, lean gains, and alternative day of fasting over the course of a month so as to get accustomed to the method that works best for you before moving to the next.

Consult with your healthcare provider before embarking on any of the fasting methods. This is strictly for anyone with any medical condition.

You are not restricted to eating a certain type or amount of food or even have to abstain from certain kinds of food when considering a fasting method. You are free to eat the food of your choice, but as far as your health and weight goals go, it is in your best interest to adhere to food rich in vegetables and fibre during the periods of eating.

Stay away from unhealthy foods during your eating days, as this helps to prevent you from accomplishing your health or weight goals. Also, drink a lot of water or other non-caloric beverages during your fast. This is so important as water helps you feel less hungry and keeps you hydrated during the periods of fasting.

Eat-stop-eat

Eat-stop-eat may not be the best method for anyone who hasn't fasted before to adopt. This method allows you to abstain from food for 24 hours at least twice a week, irrespective of the days you started out. And since abstaining from food for 24 hours would cause you to be hungrier, this method may not be right for you.

Warrior Diet happens to be the most drastic of the fasting methods as this permits you to eat very little food for 20 hours. For someone new to fasting, this method only gives you 4 hours to eat, and trying to eat a whole day's food in that short time could lead to excessive eating and a stomach upset.

Lean-gains

This permits the drinking of water while abstaining from food. A male engaging this method can last for 16 hours, then eat whatever he wants to eat the remaining 8 hours, while a female engaging this method can fast for 14 hours then eat whatever she wants to eat for the remaining 10 hours.

Alternative Day Fasting (5:2 method)

On two non-consecutive days each week, a person engaging this fast method eats up to 500 to 600 calories. People subscribe to this method to lose weight, improve their health and cholesterol levels. With this method, you are allowed to eat only the number of calories you burn each day, which in turn creates a calorie deficit leading to the loss of weight.

Be Flexible; plan ahead.

Once you get started and are getting the hang of the whole fasting thing, you can easily incorporate a short or little or no notice. Knowing that you're just starting out, it would be in your best interest to play out how your fast would proceed in at least a few days.

Endeavour that your fasting doesn't affect your family or work as this might negate the very thing your fast stands for.

Also, the place of your fast matters. Are you going to be fasting at home, during a vacation, or even in the wilderness? Let those around you know you're fasting so as to better help them be of help to you. This will save you lots of questions, especially when having a group dinner.

Understand your calorie needs

People who are considering losing weight need to create a calorie deficit for themselves. Just because there are no restrictions on your diet when you fast doesn't mean you can eat high-calorie content food.

If you are looking to gain weight, consuming more calories is what you need but if weight loss is your goal, then consume less calorie-filled food.

You can seek the counsel of a health care provider so as to know the number of required calories to be consumed daily. You can also get one of those calorie measuring kits to help you measure the intake of calories for your weight loss or gain goal.

Figure out your meal plan

Planning out your meal can help your goal of embarking on intermittent fasting, whether to lose weight or gain one. You don't have to be restrictive in your meal planning; just simply consider the place of more nutrients and a proper amount of calories in your diet.

Sticking to your calorie count and ensuring you have the needed food on hand for quick meals, cooking recipes, and snacks are a few of the benefits of planning out your meals when starting out in your fast.

Prepare for your body to feel differently.

It is perfectly normal to get a headache, feel tired or even experience shaking in your body. It is okay to feel out of sorts. These are just the negative effects of the fast taking its tolls. But after you have endured these moments as if you were going to die, you begin to experience that sense of calmness and well-being with a heightened concentration.

You also begin to experience the positive effects of the fast. Once again, your experience when starting to fast is usually negative before it gets positive, and the key to seeing it through is to put the reason (goal) for your fast before you.

Also, if you sense something is wrong beyond that feeling of tiredness, please eat something and if it persists, see your healthcare provider. You can always embark on the fast another time.

Make the calories count.

Intermittent fasting doesn't set a restriction on the number of calories consumed. Rather, it aims to help you see the nutritional value of the foods consumed. Going for food that has a high number of nutrients per calorie is highly recommended. Even though you're allowed to eat anything, practice moderation for the sake of your health.

Chapter 9: IF to weight loss

Weight reduction is the most widely recognized explanation behind individuals attempting irregular fasting. By causing you to eat fewer meals, irregular fasting can prompt a programmed decrease in calorie admission.

Studies show that discontinuous fasting can be an exceptionally incredible weight reduction apparatus. A 2014 audit study found that this eating example can cause 3–8% weight reduction or more in 3–24 weeks, which is a noteworthy sum, contrasted with most weight reduction strategies. As per a similar report, individuals additionally lost 4–7% of their midriff perimeter, showing a noteworthy loss of unsafe gut fat that develops around your organs and causes ailment.

Intermittent fasting may marginally support digestion while helping you eat fewer calories. It's an exceptionally powerful approach to shed pounds and gut fat.

Ways to Make A Fast Diet Effective

1.   Know your weight, BMI, and a waist size from the start

The waist measurement is an essential and straightforward measure of internal fat and a strong predictor of future health. People with intermittent fasting quickly lose those dangerous and unattractive centimeters. The BMI is the square of the weight (in kilograms) divided by the height (in meters). It looks ugly and may sound abstract, but it is a widely used tool to find a way to healthy weight loss. The BMI values do not take into account your body type, age, or ethnicity. You should, therefore, greet them informed. However, this is useful when you need a number.

Weigh yourself regularly. After the first phases, once a week is sufficient. If you want the numbers to drop, the morning after fasting is your best bet.

Researchers at the University of Illinois noted: "Weighing can vary significantly from food to fasting days. This weight deviation is probably due to the extra weight of food in the digestive tract.

It is not a daily change in fat mass. Future solutions may require solutions that try averaging the weight measurements on consecutive feeding and fasting days to determine weight more accurately. There are 28 tasks. If you are a person who likes structure and clarity, you may want to track your progress. Think about your goals. When and where do you want to go? Be realistic: rapid weight loss is not recommended. Please take your time. Make a plan. Write it down.

Many people recommend keeping a diet journal. Add your experience next to the number. Note the three good things that happen every day. It is a message of happiness that can be referenced over time.

2.   Find a quick friend.

You need very few accessories to be successful, but a supportive friend can be one of them. Once you are on the fast diet, tell people about it; you may find that they join you, and you will build a network of shared experiences. As the plan appeals to both men and women, couples report that doing it together is more comfortable. This way, you get mutual support, camaraderie, shared engagement, and shared anecdotes. Also, mealtimes are infinitely more comfortable if you eat with someone who understands the basics of the plot.

There are also many discussions in online discussion forums. A mum net is an excellent source of support and information. It is remarkable how reassuring it is to know that you are not alone.

3.   Quick meal preparation

Prepare your quick meal in advance, so you do not have to search for food and come across a sausage that irresistibly hides in the fridge. Keep it simple and effortlessly strive for the taste of the day. Buy and cook on nonfast days to avoid laughing at inappropriate temptations. Clean the house of junk food before embarking. It will only sing and coo in the closets, making your fasting day more difficult than it should be.

4.   Check the partial size of the calorie label.

If the serial box says "30 g", weigh it. Continue. Be surprised. Then be honest. Your calorie count is necessarily fixed and limited on an empty stomach, so it is important not to worry about how much is flowing. Here, you'll find our recommended fast food calorie counters. More importantly, do not count calories on late days.

You have better things. Wait before you eat. Resist at least 10 minutes, and preferably 15 minutes, to see if your hunger subsides (which is usually the case). If you need a snack, choose one that does not raise your insulin levels. Try carrot carrots, a handful of popcorn, apple slices, or strawberries. But do not pinch like chicken all day. Calories are stacked up quickly, and your fasting is fast. Eat consciously on a fasting day and fully absorb the fact that you are eating (especially if you have ever been in a massive traffic jam). Also, be careful with your vacation. Do not eat until you are satisfied (of course, this happens after a few weeks of practice). Find out what the concept of "satisfaction" means to you. We are all different, and it changes over time.

5.   Stay busy

"We humans are always looking for activities between meals," Leonard Cohen said. Yes, see where it takes us. So, fill your day, not your face. "No one is hungry during the first few seconds of skydiving," said Brad Pilon, the advocate of fasting. Distraction is the best defence against the dark art of the food industry, with doughnuts and nachos on every corner. If you need this doughnut, keep in mind that it will remain tomorrow.

6.   Try 2 to 2

Fast from 2:00 p.m. to 2:00 p.m., not from bedtime to bedtime. After lunch on the first day, eat modestly until late lunch on the next day.

This way, you will lose weight during sleep and will not feel uncomfortable for a day without food. This is a smart trick, but it requires a bit more focus than the all-day option. Alternatively, you can go from dinner to dinner quickly. In short, no day is fast and fun. The point is that this plan is "adapted to adjustment." Just like your waist.

Get Started

1.   Determine the start date

We strongly recommend starting on Monday. It makes more sense. After you have selected a day, you can thoroughly prepare for the start time with a few steps.

2.   Select the distribution of fast / meal to determine when to eat and fast

16/8 is recommended for beginners. You have to get used to it a lot, and it is not too difficult the first time. Select a window and decide when to stop eating the night before fasting. It will serve as a separate house. We recommend that you stick to it for the first week. After practising FI for a few weeks, it is only natural to change windows and schedules. However, it is best to keep the same time during the first week. So, if you stop eating at 9 p.m. on Sunday, you won't eat at 1 p.m. on Monday. From 1 p.m. to 9 p.m., it will be a dining room window.

3.   Spend a flirt day

Spend one day on the day before the first fast. Eat a lot and eat whatever you like. It has two purposes. First, the more foods there are in the system, the easier it is to make fast-first. Secondly, if you eat the things you want the night before, that means you won't thirst for these foods for a week.

4.   Teach people

I highly recommend talking to your loved ones about the new habits you are adopting. Explain why you do it, and why you are hired-politely informed them that you do not eat at certain times and that you will like their support, please. Warn people to make up for your chances of getting food during a fast. One of the most difficult challenges you face is that of a friend, family, or colleague who provides you with food-inform your FI and avoids it.

5.   Buy branched-chain amino acids (optional)

Branched-chain amino acids (BCAA) are beneficial on an empty stomach. These are pure forms of protein and incredibly powerful for more prolonged fasting. Consuming 10 g of BCAAs can help reduce hunger without fasting. Do not exceed 10 g per serving, but two servings are sufficient during fasting. If you want to exercise, I recommend BCAA. If you are going to exercise, we recommend that you exercise 60 minutes before and during exercise at one of the following times.

6.   Training and intermittent fasting

You do not have to exercise to take advantage of intermittent fasting. However, when you select training, you'll see unprecedented levels of results. Strength training combined with increased hormones can help you build muscle faster than expected. Lifting weights also increases the production of testosterone and growth hormone, so your body receives twice the dose of hormone production. Weight training is also very metabolic, so shred fat from your body and remember, as I said, you have more muscles, which means less fat.

I would also like to mention that strength training and exercise are probably the most effective way to protect your body from whatever the world throws at you. It has been proven to reduce stress, help with depression, increase energy levels, improve mental function, increase your happiness, improve your life, and help you live longer. Therefore, it is highly recommended to start training. If you do not have a good gym, strength exercises like pushups, squats, and lunges can help you on your journey. Finally, I would like to add one thing, if it can be speeded up, run it. I understand that planning does not mean everyone can do it, but one way to improve is to exercise and fast with a meal after exercise. Do not eat more than 2 hours after weight training, as your muscles will be disrupted, and this will negatively affect your goals.

Most women have always been passionate about keeping their bodies in shape. If you found your way here, going through this information, then you must be one of them. This is definitely great as weight regulation is a key factor in remaining healthy and reducing the risk of lifestyle diseases. Some of the conditions brought about by excess weight include:

Breathing Difficulties

When the body has excess fat, it is deposited on/in various organs, and that affects their operation. In this case, the fat in the neck interferes with the functioning of the airways, making them narrower, resulting in shallow breaths. This is especially prevalent at night when lying down, and the fat is exerting pressure on the trachea.

This could result in a condition known as sleep apnea, where breathing periodically stops then starts again. Victims tend to snore loudly and hardly feel rested even after a full night's sleep. In addition, the supply of oxygen to the brain is affected, increasing the risk of even more health conditions.

Diabetes

The extra weight increases your resistance to insulin. Research shows that up to 90% of people suffering from this type of diabetes are overweight. A decrease in weight gradually improves the intake of insulin, and eventually, some patients have been able to manage the condition with little or no medication.

Heart disease

The extra pounds make your body larger, meaning that the heart has to pump harder to take blood all around your body. Think of the heart here like an overworked machine, which wears rapidly and may eventually shut down.

Visceral fat, the one located around your abdomen, commonly known as belly fat, can also extend to surround your body organs, including the heart interfering with their functions. Even in instances where the weight does not affect the heart directly, it could cause other health conditions that raise the risk of heart disease.

High Blood Pressure

As we have established, a bigger body requires the heart to pump at a higher pressure so that the blood can reach all organs. Sustained high pressure gradually causes damage to the walls of the blood vessels. Fat and cholesterol can also collect in the inner walls of your arteries, further constricting them, and the blood will require an even higher pressure to pass through.

Overweight women double the risk of suffering from high blood pressure, while those with obesity are three times more likely to fall victim.

Fertility and Pregnancy

Excess weight makes it difficult to get pregnant and increases the chances of complications during pregnancy. The risk of high blood pressure, gestational diabetes, and preeclampsia get even higher, posing a possibly fatal risk to both the mother and the baby. In addition to these serious health conditions, excess body weight affects your self-esteem. Let us start with finding clothes; you hardly ever find something decent to wear. All the presentable dresses and tops seem tailor-made for thin women. For your remaining dignity, you choose not to squeeze into these pieces, which will leave parts of you sticking out. Eventually, you're directed to what they may call the plus-size corner, where they pack all the large dull pieces with no life at all. They actually tell you that dull colours are recommended for your size, to make you look smaller. If you actually do land some well-made clothes for big women, you'll be coughing an arm and a leg. It turns out in the fashion industry, larger women are a 'special category.'

Society is also quick to judge overweight women and often look down on them, assuming they're not good enough. Even when looking for opportunities, your body image precedes you. Have you watched those reality shows where an overweight woman came on stage, went ahead to perform, and the judges termed that as surprising? Why is it surprising? Would it have been surprising if it was a slim woman on stage? It tells you that they simply didn't expect it. An overweight woman is more often than not expected to underperform.

Even more damaging than being judged by other people is judging yourself when you don't like what you see in the mirror when you wear oversize clothes to hide your bulging sides. When you opt-out of function since you feel you will be judged. Self-judgement dents your confidence affects your performance, and it is a downward spiral from there.

Getting your weight back on track will be a starting point for so many positives in your life. Once you begin to feel good about yourself, it reflects in your attitude and demeanour. The positivity you radiate attracts similar sentiments all around you, and before you know it, your entire life is shifting for the better.

What about the Stubborn Belly Fat?
Perhaps even more frustrating than not losing weight at all is losing where you want it and not losing where you'd rather not have any. Most women do not mind some fat around the thighs, hips, and bum. In fact, that pearshaped body is much sought after in some quarters. As you grow older, however, belly fat creeps in, resulting in an apple-shaped body. Many women embark on a weight loss plan to lose this belly fat, yet it is possible to lose weight elsewhere while your belly fat stays put. The numbers on the scale are shifting, but the inches around the waist stay the same or have a negligible difference.

Other than age, belly fat has a lot to do with your feeding habits. Some foods and drinks contribute to belly fat, such as:

Soda

Sodas contain as much as 39g of sugar in a 12-ounce can. That's an entire 9.3 teaspoons of sugar! You can't imagine putting even half that amount in a similar-sized cup of tea, leave alone the entire amount. You may be avoiding eating calories, but here you're drinking them in plenty. Even those soft drinks labelled as zero sugar or diet may not be all safe. They're known to add artificial sweeteners whose end result is the same. Research has shown that the high levels of fructose in soda contributes directly to belly fat.

Fruit Juice

Thinking of what to replace the soft drinks with, fruit juice sounds like a good idea. But how much of it are you taking? Remember, the juice contains sugar as well. It may not be an artificial sweetener like in soda. But it's still sugar. It is possible to take a lot of juice as it does not have the bloating effect of gas like the one contained in soda. You're better off eating the fruits instead, and even then, go for those with less sugar. Eating fruits triggers the full signal, so you can't eat as much. They also help you load up on healthy fibre. You are taking fruits before a meal is a great way to reduce the amount of food you'll consume.

Alcohol

Regular drinkers end up with a distinct pot belly, rightfully referred to as the beer belly. That should give you a pretty good idea of where all those calories contained in alcohol end up. If you assume you're safe since you only drink occasionally, you may have to reverse that theory. Research has shown that people who drink regularly, say one or two drinks five days a week, are less likely to develop a beer belly. Those who drink quite rarely, say once a week, but take up to 10 drinks in one sitting, are at a higher risk. So if you have those 'beer nights' where you binge drink, then avoid alcohol for the rest of the week, don't be surprised if you're the first to spot a beer belly.

Trans fats

These types of fats are used in crisps and baked products such as cakes, cookies, biscuits and so on. Have you noticed that these products will stay on the shelf, without needing any refrigeration, for days or even months and still be in a good state?

The preservative here is a type of stable fat that is fortified with hydrogen. If such foods are your favourite snacks, the belly fat will creep up with time.

Carbs

Carbohydrates are an enemy to weight loss, whichever way you look at it. They digest fast, leaving you hungry and more exposed to cravings. Arrange your meals to minimize carbs while packing up with protein and vegetables.

Vegetables provide fibre, so you stay fuller for longer. Keep in mind that carbs are converted into sugar which is then converted into fats, just what you're avoiding in your weight loss journey.

Better Sleep for Better Health

Now that we've listed sleep as one of the factors affecting weight loss, let us additionally look at how it affects your health as a whole.

Most of us are getting much less than the recommended 8 hours. Even kids are staying up late doing their homework and waking up early to catch the school bus. We all seem to be in a race chasing education, careers, money, business deals and so on, and sleep is becoming a luxury we can hardly afford. It is relegated to just a few hours a day. Furthermore, we don't mind our lack of sleep; if anything, we're proud of it. We equal our lack of sleep to hard work.

However, those few (or many) hours that you're cutting from your sleep can compromise your health in the long run. They can also affect the quality of your day-to-day life. Sample these benefits that you stand to reap from sufficient sleep:

- Improved Overall Health: Several studies have revealed a link between insufficient sleep and some complex health conditions such as obesity, diabetes, heart disease, and heart attacks. In most cases, health conditions arising from lack of sleep only manifest after many years. Sleep loss will most likely not be the only cause of the condition but will contribute to aggravating it. This means that every hour of sufficient sleep that you're having now is going a long way in reducing your chances of suffering from these serious health conditions.

- Improved Weight Control: Sufficient sleep helps you maintain your ideal weight. With every hour of less sleep that you get, you increase your risk of gaining weight. With insufficient sleep comes fatigue which will make it harder for you to go through with your fast. It also causes a drop in the hormone 'leptin' which helps in making you feel full. As a result, you'll snack a lot with a particular craving for fatty foods. Are you trying to maintain your weight? Eat right, exercise and yes, sleep.

- High Productivity: When you have enough sleep, you wake up fresh and ready to work. You can concentrate more and for longer hours. With less sleep, your mood will suffer. You'll be irritable and less suitable to work in a team. Your attention span, cognition and decision making will below, and you'll have a higher risk of injury if you're working with tools and machines. If you were trying to get more work done by sleeping late, then you end up all sluggish the following day. Have you achieved your purpose? I think not. • Reduce pain: If you're suffering from acute pain as a result of an injury, a medical procedure or a health condition, getting enough sleep can make you hurt less. Sleep can actually substitute for pain relievers. Unfortunately, pain can make it difficult to sleep. In that case, you can use some sleeping pills. You now know that when in pain, you can take that nap and end up feeling better.

Those 2 or 3 extra hours of sleep really count. The above are just some of the reasons why you should turn off that TV/computer, switch off the lights and go get yourself some decent sleep. If your fasting plan is making it harder for you to sleep, try some physical exercise before bedtime. Make every effort to have a decent rest; your body will thank you for it.

Chapter 10: IF for physical healing

The type of fasting regimen should be considered alongside the physical, mental, and psychological health of the individual. Women with existing medical conditions should not combine fasting with exercises before being advised by a medical expert. So, while it is safe to practice intermittent fasting and include exercise if you are an already active person, doing so is not suitable for everyone. First of all, your metabolism can be negatively impacted if you exercise and fast for long periods. For example, if you exercise daily while fasting for more than a month, your metabolic rate can begin to slow down. Combining the two can trigger a higher rate of breaking down glycogen and body fat. This means that you burn fat at an accelerated rate. Also, when you combine these two, your growth hormones are boosted. This results in improved bone density. Your muscles are also positively impacted when you exercise. Your muscles will become more resilient to stress and age slower. This is also a quick way to trigger autophagy keeping brain cells and tissues strong, making you feel, and look younger.

Intermittent Fasting For Longevity

Another aspect of intermittent fasting that I find fascinating and innovative (excuse the term) is its anti-ageing effects and the advancements it represents for longevity. This is primarily accomplished through autophagy, which is your body's natural way of cleaning up all damaged cells and replacing them with new, healthy cells. It's like recycling. For longevity, it's fascinating.

A natural and healthy way to replace old cells and get back to producing young cells. Autophagy is programmed into us by our ancestors and works to supplement the body with energy (self-nourishment). It can't go on forever, of course, but you'll be eating every day, so your body doesn't have to go on like this forever.

Exercise Is Even Better After 50

Cardiovascular exercise is best for the heart and lungs. It improves oxygen delivery to specific parts of your body, reduces stress, improves sleep, burns fat, and improves sex drive. Some of the more common cardio exercises are running, brisk walking, and swimming. In the gym, machines such as the elliptical, treadmill, and Stairmaster are used to help with cardio. Some people are satisfied and feel like they've done enough after 20 minutes on the treadmill, but if you want to continue to be strong and independent as you grow older, you need to consider adding strength training to your workout. After 50, strength training for a woman is no longer about sixpack abs, building biceps, or vanity muscles. Instead, it has switched to maintaining a body that is healthy, strong, and is less prone to injury and illness.

Women over 50 who engage in strength training for 20 to 30 minutes a day can reap the following benefits:

- Reduced body fat: Accumulating excess body fat is not healthy for any woman at any age. To prevent many of the diseases associated with ageing, it is important to maintain healthy body weight by burning excess fat.
- Build bone density: With stronger bones, accidental falls are less likely to result in broken limbs or a visit to the emergency room. • Build muscle mass: Although you are not likely to be the next champion bodybuilder, strength training will make you an overall stronger woman who will carry herself with ease, push your lawnmower, lift your

groceries, and perform all other tasks that require you to exert some strength.

• Significant less risk of chronic diseases: In addition to keeping chronic diseases away, strength training can also reduce symptoms of some diseases you may have, such as back pain, obesity, arthritis, osteoporosis, and diabetes. Of course, the type of exercises you do if you have any chronic disease should be recommended by your doctor. • Boosts mental health: A loss of self-confidence and depression are some psychological issues that come along with ageing. Women who keep themselves fit with exercises tend to be generally more selfassured and are less likely to develop depression.

Strength Training Exercises for Women Over 50

These ten strength training exercises you can do right in the comfort of your home. All you need is a mat, a chair, and some hand weights of about 3 – 8 pounds. As you get stronger, you can increase the weight. Take a minute to rest before switching between each routine. Ensure that you move slowly through the exercises, breathe properly, and focus on maintaining the right form. If you start to feel lightheaded or dizzy during your routines, especially if you are performing the exercise during your fasting window, discontinue immediately.

Squat to Chair

This exercise is great for improving your bone health. A lot of age-related bone fractures and falls in women involve the pelvis, so this exercise will target and strengthen your pelvic bone and the surrounding muscles.

To perform this:

Stand fully upright in front of a chair as if you are ready to sit and spread your feet shoulder-width apart.

Extend your arms in front of you and keep them that way all through the movement.

Bend your knees and slowly lower your hips as if you want to sit in a chair, but don't sit. When your butt touches the chair slightly, press into your heels to get back your initial standing position; repeat that about 10 to 15 times.

Forearm Plank

This exercise targets your core and shoulders.

Here's how to do it:

Get into a push-up position, but with your arms bent at the elbows such that your forearm is supporting your weight.

Keep your body off the mat or floor and keep your back straight at all times. Don't raise or drop your hips. This will engage your core. Hold the position for 30 seconds and then drop to your knees. Repeat ten times.

Modified Push-ups

This routine targets your arms, shoulders, and core.

How's how to do it:

Kneel on your mat. Place your hands on the mat below your shoulders and let your knees be behind your hips so that your back is stretched at an angle.

Tuck your toes under and tighten your abdominal muscles. Gradually bend your elbows as you lower your chest toward the floor.

Push back on your arms to press your chest back to your previous position. Repeat as many times as is comfortable.

Bird Dog

When done correctly, this exercise can strengthen the muscles of your posterior chain as it targets your back and core. It may seem easy at first but can be a bit tricky.

To do this correctly:

Go on all fours on your mat.

Tighten your abdominal muscles and shift your weight to your right knee and left hand. Ensure that both your hands and legs are extended as far as possible and stay in that position for about 5 seconds. Return to your starting position. This is one repetition. Switch to your left knee and right hand and repeat the movement. Alternate between both sides for 20 repetitions.

Shoulder Overhead Press

This targets your biceps, shoulders, and back.

To perform this move:

With dumbbells in both hands, stand and spread your feet shoulder-width apart.

Bring the dumbbells up to the sides of your head and tighten your abdominal muscles.

Slowly return to the first position. Repeat ten times.

Chest Fly

This targets your chest, back, core, and glutes.

To do this:

Lie with your back flat on your mat, your knees at an angle close to 90 degrees, and your feet firmly planted on the floor or mat.

Hold dumbbells in both hands over your chest. Keep your palms facing each other and gently open your hands away from your chest. Let your upper arms touch the floor without releasing the tension in them.

Contract your chest muscles and slowly return the dumbbells to the initial position. Repeat about ten times.

Standing Calf Raise

This exercise improves the mobility of your lower legs and feet and also improves your stability.

Here's how to perform it.

Hold a dumbbell in your left hand and place your right hand on something sturdy to give you balance.

When you are sure of your balance, lift your left foot off the floor with the dumbbell hanging at your side. Stand erect and move your weight such that you are almost standing on your toes.

Single-Leg Hamstring Bridge

This move targets your glutes, quads, and hamstrings.

Place your arms flat by your side and lift one leg straight.

Contract your glutes as you lift your hips into a bridge position with your arms still in position. Hold for about 2 to 3 seconds and drop your hips to the mat. Repeat about ten times before switching your leg. Do the same again.

Bent-Over Row

This targets your back muscles and spine.

To do this:

Hold dumbbells in both hands and stand behind a sturdy object (for example, a chair). Bend forward and rest your head on the chosen object. Relax your neck and slightly bend your knees. With both palms facing each other pull, the dumbbells to touch your ribs. Hold the position for about 2 to 5 seconds and slowly return to the starting position. Repeat 10 to 15 times.

Basic Ab

A distended belly is a common occurrence in older women. This exercise can strengthen and tighten the abdominal muscles bringing them inward toward your spine.

To perform this:

Lie on your back with your feet firmly planted on the floor and your knees bent. Relax your upper body and rest your hands on your thighs.

As you exhale, lift yourself upward off the mat or floor. Stop the upward movement when your hands are resting on your knees. Hold the position for about 2 to 5 seconds and then slowly return to the starting position. Repeat for about 20 to 30 times.

Chapter 11: Foods to eat & avoid

During intermittent fasting, feeding is more about being healthy than simply losing weight quickly. Thus, selecting nutrient-dense foods such as veggies, fruits, lean proteins, and healthy fats is critically important.

The list of intermittent fasting foods should include:

1. PROTEIN

Dietary Allowance (RDA) for protein. Depending on your health objectives and level of operation, your requirements can differ.

By reducing energy consumption, increasing satiety, and improving metabolism, protein helps you lose weight.

Besides, increased protein consumption helps create muscle when paired with strength training. As muscle burns more calories than fat, having more muscle in the body naturally increases the metabolism.

A recent study indicates that having more muscle in your legs will help reduce the development of belly fat in healthy men.

The IF food list for protein include:

• Poultry and fish

• Seafood

• Eggs

• Beans and legumes

• Soy

• Seeds and nuts
• Whole grains

2. CARBS

45 to 65 per cent of the daily calories should come from carbohydrates, according to the Dietary Recommendations for Americans (carbs).

Carbs are the main source of your body's nutrition. The other two are fat and protein. Carbs come in different ways. Sugar, carbohydrate, and starch are the most notable among them.

Carbs for causing weight gain also get a poor rap. Not all carbohydrates, however, are produced equally and are not necessarily fattening.

Make sure that foods high in fibre and starch but low in sugar are selected.

A 2015 study indicates that consuming 30 grams of fibre every day will lead to weight loss, glucose levels improving, and blood pressure decreasing.

It isn't an uphill struggle to get 30 grams of fibre from your diet. By consuming a basic egg sandwich, Mediterranean barley with chickpeas, peanut butter apple, and enchiladas with chicken and black peas, you will get them.

The IF food list for carbs include:

• Sweet potatoes

• Quinoa

• Oats

• Beetroots

• Brown rice
• Mangoes

• Apples

- Berries

- Bananas

- Kidney beans

- Pears

- Carrots

- Broccoli

- Brussels sprouts

- Avocado

- Almonds

- Chickpeas

- Chia seeds

3. FATS

Fats should contribute 20 per cent to 35 per cent of your daily calories, according to the 2015-2020 Dietary Recommendations for Americans. Most significantly, saturated fat does not account for more than 10% of daily calories.

Fats, depending on the form, maybe good, poor, or simply in-between.

Trans fats, for example, increase inflammation, decrease "good cholesterol levels, and increase "bad cholesterol levels. They are found in fruit and baked goods that are fried.

Saturated fats can raise the risk of heart disease. Expert views on this, however, vary. Eating them in moderation is wise. High levels of saturated fats are present in red meat, whole milk, coconut oil, and baked goods.

The monounsaturated and polyunsaturated fats provide healthy fats. These fats can reduce the risk of heart disease, decrease blood pressure, and decrease fat levels in the blood.

The rich sources of these fats include olive oil, peanut oil, canola oil, safflower oil, sunflower oil, and soybean oil.

The IF food list for fats include:

• Avocados

• Cheese

• Nuts

• Whole eggs

• Dark chocolate

• Chia seeds

• Fatty fish

• Full-fat yoghurt

• Extra virgin olive oil (EVOO)

4. For a HEALTHY GUT

An increasing body of evidence suggests that the secret to your overall wellbeing is your intestinal health. Your intestine has billions of bacteria known as microbiota in its home.
These bacteria impair your gut health, digestion, and mental health. In many chronic disorders, they can also play a critical role.

Therefore, particularly when you are fasting intermittently, you should take care of those tiny bugs in your stomach.

The intermittent fasting food list for a healthy gut include:

• All vegetables

• Kefir

• Fermented vegetables

• Kimchi

• Miso

• Sauerkraut

• Kombucha

• Tempeh

These foods will also help you lose weight, in addition to keeping your gut safe by:

• Reducing fat absorption from the gut.

• Increasing the excretion via stools of ingested fat.

• Reducing the consumption of calories.

5. HYDRATION

The daily fluid requirement, according to the National Academies of Sciences, Engineering, and Medicine, is:

About 3.7 litres (15.5 cups) for men.
About 2.7 litres (11.5 cups) for women.

Fluids include water, as well as water-containing foods and beverages.

During intermittent fasting, remaining hydrated is important for your health. Headaches, extreme tiredness, and dizziness may be caused by dehydration.

Dehydration can make these side effects of fasting worse or even extreme if you are still dealing with them.

The intermittent fasting food list for hydration include:

• Water

• Black coffee or tea

• Sparkling water

• Watermelon

• Cantaloupe

• Peaches

• Strawberries

• Oranges

• Lettuce

• Cucumber

• Skim milk

• Celery

• Plain yoghurt

• Tomatoes

Interestingly, drinking a lot of water will help with weight loss as well. A study reviewed in 2016 reports that proper hydration will help you lose weight through:

They are decreasing appetite or consumption of food.

Rising burning of fat.

FOR FATS (75% OF YOUR DAILY CALORIES)

• Nuts

• Cheese

• Avocados

• Whole eggs

• Dark chocolate

• Chia seeds

• Extra virgin olive oil (EVOO)

• Fatty fish

• Full-fat yoghurt

FOR PROTEIN (20% OF YOUR DAILY CALORIES)

• Eggs

• Poultry and fish

• Seafood

• Seeds and nuts

• Soy
• Beans and legumes

• Whole grains

FOR CARBS (5% OF YOUR DAILY CALORIES)

• Beetroots

• Sweet potatoes

- Quinoa

- Brown rice

- Oats

The food list for intermittent fasting vegetarian diet includes:

FOR PROTEIN

- Seeds and nuts

- Beans and legumes

- Whole grains

- Soy

FOR CARBS

- Beetroots

- Sweet potatoes

- Quinoa

- Brown rice

- Bananas

- Oats
- Mangoes

- Apples

- Kidney beans

- Pears

- Berries

- Carrots

- Broccoli

- Brussels sprouts

- Avocado

- Almonds

- Chickpeas

- Chia seeds

FOR FATS

- Nuts

- Cheese

- Avocados

- Chia seeds

- Full-fat yoghurt

- Dark chocolate

- Extra virgin olive oil (EVOO) **Superfoods to Eat for Women Over 50 In Intermittent Fasting Avocado**

Eating the highest-calorie food when attempting to lose weight can seem strange. Although, because of its high content of unsaturated fat, avocados can make you feel full throughout the day, even the longest times of fasting. Even when a person doesn't feel full, evidence shows unsaturated fats help hold your body feel full. The body sends signals that it has adequate calories and will not move into hunger mode in an emergency. Unsaturated fats hold these signals running for longer, even though you get a little hungry during a fasting time. Another research also showed that it could keep you satisfied for hours. so you must add these green mushy fruit to your diet during intermittent fasting

Fish & Seafood

There is a cause that the Nutritional Recommendations suggest that two or three servings of 4 ounces of fish be consumed each week. It includes sufficient quantities of vitamin D, besides being high in good fats and protein. If you eat during fasting with small windows, don't you want to eat nutrition-packed food. There are many ways to enjoy fish that one can never run out of ideas.

Cruciferous Vegetables

Broccoli, cauliflower, and Brussels sprouts are full of the most important nutrition fibre. It's essential to consume fibre-rich foods that keep the body regular and make the gut function smoothly, especially when you eat after intervals. Fibre may also help one to feel full, which might be a positive thing if you can't eat for 16 hours. Cruciferous vegetables may also minimize cancer risk.

Potatoes

As mentioned before, potatoes are one of the heartiest food to eat, that will keep you full, as the main course or snack or in lunch during intermittent fasting. But French fries and potato chips do not count as healthy options.

Legumes & Beans

In the IF lifestyle, the favourite addition to chilli maybe your best mate. Food, including carbohydrates, offers energy for physical activity. It is not asked of you to carb-load to insane amounts, but tossing some low-calorie carbohydrates like legumes and beans into the diet plan will certainly not cause any harm. During the fasting hours, this will hold you active, and without calorie limits, foods such as black beans, chickpeas, peas, and lentils are shown to lower body weight.

Probiotics

Do you know what good bacteria want the most in the gut? Diversity & consistency. That implies that when they are hungry, they aren't content. And you can feel certain annoying side effects, including constipation, while the stomach isn't content. Add probiotic-rich products such as kefir, sauerkraut, and Kombucha to the diet to combat this discomfort.

Eggs

6.24 grams of protein is provided by one big egg and cooked up in minutes. And it is important to get as much protein as needed to sustain fullness and build muscle, particularly when one eats less. Women who had an egg breakfast rather than a bagel are far less hungry and ate less during the day, a 2010 study showed. In other terms, why not hard-boil those eggs while you're hunting for anything to do during the fasting period? And, when the time is perfect, you should enjoy them.

Whole Grains

It appears like going on a diet and consuming carbohydrates fit in two separate buckets. To realize that this is not necessarily the case, you'll be super happy. Whole grains supply plenty of nutrition and fibre, but eating less goes a long way to keep yourself full. So do not hold back from wholegrain like bulgar, farro, bulgur, spelt, Kamut, amaranth, millet, freekeh, or sorghum, from your comfort place.

Foods to Avoid During Intermittent Fasting

You can keep away from foods that contain huge amounts of salt, sugar, and fat that are calorie-dense. These foods won't fill you up fast, and they might also leave you hungry. They have little or no nutrients, as well.

Avoid these ingredients to sustain a safe intermittent feeding regimen:

- Processed foods
- Snack chips.
- Refined grains
- Trans-fat
- Alcoholic beverages
- Sugar-sweetened beverages
- Microwave popcorn.
- Candy bars
- Processed meat

In addition, you must avoid foods that are rich in added sugar. Sugar is devoid of any nutrients and contributes to sweet, hollow calories in the form of refined foods and beverages, which is what you should avoid while you're intermittently fasting. Because the sugar metabolizes super-fast, it will make you even hungrier.

You should avoid these sugar-packed foods if you are trying to do intermittent fasting:

- Frosted Cakes.
- Cookies
- Sugar added Fruit juice.
- Candies
- Sugary cereals and granola

- Barbecue sauce and ketchup.

Foods such as nuts, lean proteins, seeds, fresh vegetables, and fruits should be your main focus during intermittent fasting as they help in weight loss and help keep your stomach full.

To prevent any nutritional deficiencies, healthy eating is the key to successful intermittent fasting.

Chapter 12: Mistakes to avoid during IF

Searching for an Excessive Number of Improvements Too Fast

You are planning to start something new, and you are anxious to get all the awards as fast as anyone might think possible. It is simply normal that you are amped up for this new way of life and you need to completely jump into it. By the by, endeavoring to quickly get a particular number of enhancements too soon may disturb your undertakings.

The key is to start step by step with a few changes in a steady progression. For example, in the event that you have decided to do 2 500-calorie days consistently while having an ordinary measure of calories the other 5; think about starting with just 1 single 500-calorie day. After a long time, you will feel more sure including the second day into your week after week plan.

Not Taking Care of Your Hydration

Remaining in a fasting state can be testing whether or not you are not eating. Most beverages will break the fast and exceptionally decrease any advantages. Notwithstanding the way that they are fat and calorie-free, it is definitely not keen to drink "diet" soda pops. Undoubtedly, even sugars that have 0 calories can contrarily impact your insulin levels.

Mistaking Thirst for Hunger

While it is critical not to drink wrong liquids when fasting, it is comparably fundamental to guarantee you drink enough water. Not getting enough water can make you hungry, and it is definitely not hard to now and then mistake hunger for hunger.

Individuals get a lot of water from a decent piece of the food sources they eat.

Overall food information expresses that 20% of the water our bodies use starts from food. This suggests that on the off chance that you are not eating for a couple of hours you should drink around 20% more water than expected to make up for any shortage.

Eating Unhealthy Foods

Since intermittent fasting isn't for the most part a diet plan, there are no food sources that are "illegal." This can lead numerous individuals to fall into the catch of gorge on shoddy nourishment the second their fasting is up and the eating time opens. Do whatever it takes not to make a propensity for unfortunate eating imagining that fasting will make up for it.

Cause a summary of the multitude of solid food sources you to do appreciate. Do customary looking for food and attempt to adhere to your food choices. While satisfying your craving with not actually solid bites here and there can be okay, for ideal well-being and weight reduction accomplishment, it is critical to eat as healthy as conceivable in light of the current situation. Eating the correct nourishment is essential to exploiting any weight-reduction plan. Nourishments plentiful in calcium, protein, and nutrient B-12 ought to be high on your staple rundown, especially for ladies more than 50.

Indulging After Each Fast

This is probably the best snare for the 2 novices and individuals who have been fasting intermittently for a long time. Rehearsing intermittent fasting to get more fit will lose viability in the event that you wind up taking in an exorbitant measure of calories on each possibility you need to eat.

One way to deal with keep away from indulging is to eat bigger measures of better nourishments during your eating window. This would incorporate loads of solid plates of blended greens and fresh vegetables. It is also a shrewd plan to orchestrate meals and having flavors arranged before your fast period begins. Subsequently, you are not enticed to simply get anything. Recollect that it can take as long as around 14 days until you have changed and adjusted to the point that you won't feel that ravenous after each fasting period.

Attempting to Stick to the Wrong Plan

There is a wide range of ways to deal with put intermittent fasting into your day-by-day plan. For example, if your fasting plan incorporates not eating from 8 p.m. until early evening each day and you have a difficult action that starts directly in the initial segment of the day, this is in all probability not the right arrangement for you.

To get the most prizes of intermittent fasting, you should take as much time as is needed to altogether investigate various sorts of plans. It is OK in the event that it takes somewhat more to discover the arrangement that best works for you.

Working Out Too Much or Too Little

It is basic to stay as unique as could be expected, yet you would not really like to exaggerate, particularly during your fasting times. A couple of novices may feel overpowered, starting to follow another eating plan, and may neglect practice through and through. Others may be excited to the point that they wind up trying too hard.

It is a keen idea to pick a moderate exercise plan, especially when starting. Walking the pooch for 20 minutes or riding your bike to work are basic ways to deal with add moderate exercise to your standard schedule.

Not Drinking Enough Water
Perhaps quite possibly the most widely recognized and effectively avoidable intermittent fasting botches isn't taking in enough water.

We realize that drinking water is principal for general well-being, obviously, yet it is much more critical when you are fasting.

Why? Since more often than not when we feel hungry, we are really got dried out.

Would you be able to envision how your appetite may be impacted by the absence of water when you are attempting to experience the fundamental piece of the day without eating?

Sneaking more water into your day is just about as straightforward as several fundamental changes.

A couple of individuals really are exhausted drinking plain water. Trust me, one thing that might be a good thought is to 2–3 Mio Drops (or other water enhancers) to water. It will have a colossal impact!

Misconstruing Real Hunger Signs

Maybe the best thing that I have gained from my intermittent fasting test is that I found a decent speed about when hunger shows.

It doesn't come at 9 a.m., the point at which I have been wakeful for 1 hour and last ate a late-night snack at 11 p.m. the earlier evening.

However, once more, you are not actually ravenous.

Intermittent fasting will instruct you that on the off potential for success that you have by fasting sufficiently long, as a rule, your "hunger" will obscure commonly in close to 5–10 minutes.

How often grinding away you were wanting to go to eat, at that point a few nonetheless, some very late surge work appeared, and 1–2 hours cruised by, while you ignored your stomach's dissent?

What before resembled the direst need, eating, was dominated by something new that sprung up. What's more, you endure!

Regardless, yielding and eating too soon is one of the genuine misunderstandings with intermittent fasting. Feel that essentially drinking some water and permitting it ten minutes or somewhere in the vicinity, you will, for the most part, your hunger will quiet down.

Make an effort not to break your intermittent fasting plan before you even start.

Do whatever it takes not to effectively yield to false yearning!

Blaming Intermittent Fasting to Overeat

Quite possibly the most unsafe intermittent fasting botches is yield to the impulse to say, "What the hell, I have starved myself all through all the day, I have the right to remunerate myself for dinner!" and afterward making a plunge an insane dining experience of shoddy nourishment bombarding yourself with unfortunate stuff.

Kindly don't be that lady.

You would feel miserable and probably put-on weight.

We don't need that.

Notwithstanding the way that intermittent fasting isn't a diet since it doesn't restrict what you eat, it is yet basic to make better food choices. You need a large portion of all to have a healthy connection with your food and your body.

You can totally gorge and put-on weight even by eating just once each day, on the off chance that you are eating a more prominent number of calories than your body burns-through.

Not Eating Enough

All things considered, for certain individuals, not eating for an especially significant period, it's not bizarre to turn out to be less ravenous.

Now and again, fasting can completely execute your craving.

Except if you are intentionally doing an absolute fast (not proposed if not under clinical control), nonetheless, it is definitely not rather a smart thought to choose not to eat enough.

On the off chance that you ought not to eat adequately for a really long time, you can undoubtedly wreck your assimilation and unbalance your chemicals.

Besides, you will keep your body from getting principal supplements, which can help your well-being evading issues that are undeniably more significant than passing several extra pounds.

Counsel your doctor about a total, sound calorie consumption that is good for weight reduction and may help you arrive at your ideal results.

Neglecting to Plan Your Meals in Advance

While calorie counting isn't significant (anyway genuinely, you will give more indications of progress results in the event that you do it), cautiously arranging and pondering what you will eat when your eating period shows up is an incredible intermittent fasting hack.

This will permit you not to need to extemporize when you are at long last going to take a seat at the table.

As opposed to going like "I'm starving and need to eat now regardless" and afterward making a beeline for the nearest, least expensive, and more unfortunate shoddy nourishment, you better figure out how to advise yourself "indeed, I'm feeling hungry now, yet I can pause, I'm not kicking the bucket and something solid and delectable is hanging tight for me, later."

Using this chance to consider what you will eat when you eat and adhering to better choices will just have benefits for you over the long haul.

You will figure out how to eat for compelling weight reduction, while diminishing caloric admission, keeping you fulfilled, and boosting your fearlessness.

In the event that you are fasting for 16 hours, you can undoubtedly contribute 5 minutes of your opportunity to arrange for what meal will break your fast later.

Not Exercising at All

While the facts confirm that you really could, regardless, lose a great deal of weight with intermittent fasting even without working out by any means, why in the world would you leave behind the amazing opportunity to lose fundamentally more, faster, and with a lot of different advantages for your well-being?

It truly has absolutely no explanation.

Time can't avoid being time. A month is a month. If in 1 month you could be sluggish and shed 5 pounds or exercise 3 times each week and lose 10, wouldn't you go for the 10?

Chapter 13: Exercises to do during IF

Maintaining physical activity past the age of 50 years will enable you to:

- Preserve lean muscle and bone mass
- Achieve or maintain a healthy body weight
- Maintain high levels of your energy
-

Increase strength, flexibility, as well as the ability to perform your tasks every day

- Reduce stress, anxiety, and depression
- Slow down the decline in your body that is usually associated with age

As much as you would want to follow the advice to maintaining your health past the age of 50, you should endeavour to engage in workout exercises that you enjoy because they could keep you from quitting.

Fasting will help you lose weight and just remain slim, but if you want some muscle, then exercise will avail you of that. The reduced calorie intake in your diet will give you similar results as exercise – weight loss. However, there are so many other benefits you'll get from exercising that you may not get from the fast or will get them at a lower level.

Reduce Stress

Physical exercise provides a positive distraction from the conflict that is taking place in your mind causing you stress. It has a calming, relaxing effect. Though tiring at first, exercise quickly evolves into fun as the adrenalin kicks in and you just want to keep going. Choose something that you enjoy. It could be walking, jogging, running, cycling, swimming or even dancing. Yes, just pop in a tune and dance around the house till you're all sweaty! Then take a relaxing dip in the tub. By the time you step out of the shower, you'll have a hard time recalling what was stressing you up. Also related to reduced stress is the quality of sleep. Stress messes up your sleep; you toss and turn for the better part of the night and wake up without having had any meaningful rest. Schedule some exercises in the evening for improved sleep. Stress and poor sleep both negatively affect your ability to fast. Managing them through exercise allows you to have an easier fast.

Boosts Energy Levels

For the first few moments of the exercise, you'll feel some fatigue, then the endorphins check-in and your energy levels surge. There are those who will exercise in the morning so that they can be energized for the rest of the day. In the long term, exercise contributes to building muscle which makes the body stronger. If you're having one of those sluggish days, even taking a few stretches at your desk makes you feel better. This will come in handy when you're experiencing low energy levels during a fast.

Accelerates Weight Loss

By exercising, you complement the weight loss abilities of intermittent fasting. The body in a fasted state, past the fifth hour when all the food in the system has been used up, turns to the fat deposits for energy. The higher the energy demands, the more calories you burn. When you exercise during this phase, you increase the energy demands many times over. More calories are burnt to meet energy needs. By the end of the session, you lose a significantly higher amount of fat compared to when fasting only. If you accompany every fasting session with a form of exercise, you will lose weight much faster compared to those relying on the fast alone.

Muscle Gain

You can exercise during the eating period or the fasting period. In the case above, exercising takes place during the fasting period, and the result is weight loss. On the other hand, exercising during the eating period causes muscle gain. Exercise ensures that the food eaten goes on to build muscle as opposed to being stored as fat.

Exercise is Fun

Physical activity should be that part of your day that you look forward to. Join in with others with similar interests and exercise together. You will form new friends and probably find a new community (even online) to engage with. Even in instances when you're are alone, such as when you have to exercise indoors, you still end up in a better mood.

Improve Sex

We have already seen that your energy is increased by exercise. Your sex life will also benefit from this energy. In addition, most people find vigorous physical activity arousing.

That's like foreplay already done for you. Eventually, exercise leads to an improved body image. Feeling more attractive does wonder for your sex life.

Prevent and Manage Lifestyle Diseases

Most chronic diseases are brought about by poor diet and inactivity, which results in excess weight. When you exercise, you're already a step ahead in lowering the risk factors of diseases like high blood pressure, type 2 diabetes, heart disease, obesity, and arthritis.

Even when living with such a disease, making an effort to remain active makes it easier to manage. Here intermittent fasting and exercise complement each other perfectly.

Do Women need muscle?

When we talk of building muscle, the most common image in mind is that of ripped bodybuilders with their muscles bulging all over the place. This is not the muscle we're talking about here, at least not to that extent. Won't muscles make you look masculine? Again, this is a matter of quantity. Here we aim to promote the formation of lean skeletal muscle, one that will help you move with ease without bulging through your clothes. Such muscle adds to your strength, so you find it easier to perform your everyday activities. You no longer have to call for help every time you want to move/lift the slightest thing in the house. Muscles also boost metabolism and prevent glucose from being stored as fat. You will end up with a fit, toned look, the kind you'd be proud to show off in a bikini.

If fitting exercise into your schedule is a challenge, one of the best devices that you can get is a treadmill. It allows you to exercise any time from the comfort of your house. Running on the treadmill for an hour or so every day while in the fasted state will help burn even more fat, thus lose more weight.

6 Tips to Maximize your Treadmill Runs

Running on the treadmill is a great alternative to outdoor running. From a distance, running on a treadmill looks super easy; you just hop on and start running, right? Not so fast! Excuse the pun. If you do so without understanding the parameters of the treadmill and how they affect your running, you might not get the most from the exercise.

Start Slow
Just as with any other exercise routine, you need to start with a warm-up. With a treadmill, it is tempting to just set the speed and hit the speed right away. A warm-up increases body temperature, making it easier for muscles to contract and relax. Such flexible muscles prepare the body for faster movement and reduce the chances of an injury. Start with minimum speed and walk/jog for 5-10 minutes.

Check the Incline

If you're just starting out or getting back to running after a long break, you can leave the treadmill at zero inclines as you build your form. Then set the incline to 1-2%. This is the best incline for sustained indoor running since there's no wind resistance. Vary the incline without exceeding 7%.

Combine steep with flat running. Changing the incline gives you variation, just as you'd experience when running outside.

Posture

Maintain an upright posture without leaning forward. It's tempting to keep looking down to see how much time or distance you've covered. To avoid this, you can visualize a running route that you're familiar with. Keep your head up and your arms swinging. Avoid holding onto the handrail; it is only supposed to assist you when getting on and off the treadmill and in the rare case of an injury while running.

Stride

Aim for short, quick steps as opposed to long strides. Aim to strike the surface mid-foot. A long stride makes you strike heel-first, which can leave you with pain around the ankles. Work on increasing your steps per minute. Elite runners can go as high as 180. You might be far from that, but you can steadily work your way up, especially if you're practising for racing purposes.

Hydrate

You may be surprised that you actually sweat more on the treadmill compared to the outdoors, where the wind keeps you cool. Keep your water bottle close. It is actually easier to hydrate on the treadmill as you don't have to bear the weight of carrying the water bottle as you run.

Cool Down

At the end of your run, cool down before you come off the treadmill. Reduce the speed gradually and spend the last 5 minutes jogging or walking. This will not only prevent dizziness but also keep you from injury associated with coming off a moving treadmill.

Advantages of Running on a Treadmill

Buying a simple treadmill for your home is one of the best investments that you can make for your health. The alternative, of course, is to run outside, which you may argue you can easily do for free. However, running on the treadmill has several benefits. Consider the following:

Great for Beginners

Treadmill running is easier on the body, which is essential for starters and those getting back to exercising after a prolonged break. The padded surface of the treadmill provides a smoother and softer surface for landing, which absorbs the impact better compared to concrete or bare earth. Unlike the outdoors, you can control gradient throughout, so you don't have to deal with strenuous, steep runs just yet. No Worries about the Weather Weather elements often disrupt the outdoor exercise. Rain, scorching sun, fog can make your run difficult if not impossible. Given that such unfavourable weather sometimes goes on for months, your schedule will be disrupted immensely. The option of running indoors protects you from such interruptions. Time is also of the essence here. With a treadmill, you can run any time; early morning, midday or even at night. Lack of time will no longer be an excuse when you have the machine in the house.

You can simulate a race.

Should you want to train for a race, you can simulate the race conditions so that your body can acclimatize in good time. You can create conditions that may not be available where you live but will be present in the race. Setting the treadmill on an incline helps you prepare for hills. Furthermore, you run uphill without having to run downhill, as would be the case if you were running outside. You can set the room temperature to match the one you're expecting at the race. This is also an opportunity to test your new running outfit and shoes and avoid any unpleasant surprises at the race.

Safety

The outdoors is always unpredictable, especially if your area does not have designated walking/running tracks. You have to jostle for space with other people and even cars. This slows you down, and the chances of an injury are high. If you normally walk/run around when listening to music from your earphones, you're even at a higher risk since you may not hear a car/bike hoot or someone shouting at you to get out of the way. Running indoors eliminates such hassle and ensures your running is safe.

Pace Control
A treadmill makes it easy to track the parameters of your running. Once you set the time/mileage, you can track the distance you have covered, how long it has taken, the time/distance you have left, etc. If you're getting ready for a race, you can easily keep tabs on your progress and determine if you're accomplishing your goals.

You can have your meal right.

If you prefer to exercise at the very end of your fasting period, then exercising at home allows you to grab a meal right away. If your fast ends and you're out there, you may be tempted to eat whatever is at hand to satiate your hunger which is now at its peak. At home, you can be assured that you're getting a healthy meal and not jeopardizing the benefits of the fast.

If you find indoor running monotonous, try to spice it up by listening to music or an audiobook. Some even watch TV while running.

You can also alternate with a different workout routine. Enjoy the convenience as you reap the benefits of running and keeping fit.

Try Yoga; at Zero Budget

This is another great exercise regime that is largely zero-cost. Yoga is mostly associated with mental wellness, as it involves quiet time and meditation. However, it has several physical benefits as well. If you're seeking to keep fit or even lose weight, consider including Yoga sessions in your routine. Unlike exercising in the gym or even outdoor, you can practice yoga in any space.

Anywhere

You don't need any machinery, equipment or a vast space. The main component of Yoga is just you. Even the mat is not compulsory. You can work out on your usual carpet at home, or better still, outside on the grass. Don't you have workout clothes or shoes? No problem! Just pick any comfortable clothes and shoes from your wardrobe. You can even go barefoot. Simply get into position and strike your poses.

Full Body Workout

The versatile nature of Yoga allows you to stretch every part of the body. In the beginning, you'll be forgiven for striking simple poses, but as you go along, you can attempt more challenging ones. Experienced Yoga masters are like contortionists; they can easily twist and turn every joint in their body. Regular yoga will not only relax your mind, but your body will also be well toned.

Zero Competition

Group workouts have this silent competition, each trying to outdo the others. Gyms are probably the most vicious in this disguised rivalry. From those running on the treadmill, lifting weights to those doing press-ups, there is always that side-eye to see if the neighbour is doing it better. Or faster. If you're out of shape, this scenario is nothing but intimidating. Many people detest the gym for this very reason. With Yoga, you do your thing. Even in group sessions, each is too engrossed in their own moves to notice what the next is doing. You can move at your own pace and style and get the best from the routine.

Variety

Yoga involves a vast spectrum of poses and probably, even more, are being introduced as we speak. You do not have to keep following the same routine. You can mix up the moves, twists, and turns so that your session is unique each time. While at it, feel free to devise some new moves, so your sessions will always have that unique twist to prevent monotony.

Minimal Injury

Sustaining an injury during yoga is almost unheard of. Provided you don't push yourself too hard, and you don't have a significant previous injury, you can be assured of practising yoga with no injuries. The fact that you're not using any machinery or equipment makes further distances Yoga from injury.

Light Enough for Fasting Period

If your energy levels are limited during the fasting period, and you're looking for a form of exercise with the least strain, then yoga is just the one for you. You can strike the simple movements comfortably and still manage to burn some calories in the process.

No matter how tiny your space is, Yoga is always an option. Your office, sitting room, bedroom, backyard and any other can easily host your sessions. Time and financial constraints should be no longer a hindrance; all you need is you.

Cycling is also a great option, especially if you're just getting into strength training. It's not only fun; it also keeps you fit, helps you lose weight and improve your overall cardiovascular health. You can cycle indoors on a stationary bike or a normal bike outdoors.

If you're just starting out, go for a stationary bike if you have that option. Here you can cycle without worrying about accidents. Stationary bikes are also recommended if you're out of shape since most of their parameters are adjustable. You can have back support as well. You start cycling at a low resistance then progress with time.

Indoor bikes allow you to exercise any time, without worrying about the weather, harsh terrain or accidents. However, they're bound to get boring with time since they confine you to the same environment, which gets monotonous with time. The ultimate goal should be to venture out and ride as you enjoy the sights and sounds of nature.

Once you've built your endurance to a reliable level, you can proceed to outdoor cycling. Shop for the right bike for your body size. The seat, pedals, and handlebars should be comfortable to reach. Depending on the terrain in your area, you can go for a mountain, road or cruising bike.

In the beginning, concentrate on getting the balance right. Master the riding technique to avoid falls and related accidents. Flat, even surfaces work best for new riders. If you have a cycling track where you live, you're lucky.

Once you get the hang of it, you can venture out to more challenging tracks. Time yourself while at it, and strive to get faster each time.

Pay attention to the safety gear. Start with the cycling helmet. Then there are the safety pads for the elbows and knees. In case of an incident, these should protect you from the impact.

Riding improves many facets of your life;

- It is a low impact exercise compared to walking or running. You get to exercise safely without putting too much pressure on the knees and ankles. Good for you if you're overweight and want to lose calories without straining your joints.

-
- Cycling helps you build leg muscles making your legs stronger for walking or running.
- It saves you time when you ride to work or for other errands. You get to avoid the traffic jams, save the time that you could have spent waiting for the train/bus and eliminate the stress of looking for a parking spot.
- You can establish new networks by joining a cycling group where you meet new people, engage in new activities and go to places you probably never have ventured into on your own.

Will you prefer riding in the fasted state or in the fed state? That depends on your needs. If you're majorly concentrating on shedding weight, then cycling when fasted will help you burn more calories. Cycling in your fed state, on the other hand, will contribute to lean muscle on the arms and legs.

Exercise in Outdoors More

Even when you have access to a gym, or have a treadmill in the house, once in a while, make that deliberate effort to exercise outdoors. Nature is simply unbeatable and presents plenty of elements that even the most sophisticated gym cannot.

Savour the Nature

After spending most of your days indoors, in the office, home, even shopping malls, how about you spend some time outdoors when working out? Enjoy the sights and sounds, the fresh air, invigorating in the sunshine. Get some much-needed Vitamin D for your bones.

Reduce Stress

To keep your fasting on track, one of the things you have to keep at bay or at least manage is stress. Stress often leads to binge eating of comfort food, something you should avoid at all cost. It disrupts the hormones leaving you fighting hunger pangs for the better part of the fast. Ideally, the hunger pangs should be minimally disruptive. Stress also affects your quality of sleep, and once you're not well-rested, even your fasting ability is jeopardized. Exercising outside in the vast nature gives you a positive distraction from your stress and leaves you more relaxed.

New Scenery

Exercising outdoors gives you an opportunity to exercise in a new location each time. Whether you're in your backyard, the park, or a nature trail, the outdoors always has something to offer.

Trade your treadmill running/walking for a session in the park or any other nature trail of your choice. Watch the sunrise as you jog. Run under the shades of the trees with birds chirping overhead, taking in all that fresh air. Look for new places to walk/run/cycle. By the end of the sessions, you'll have so much more than toned muscles.

Space

The outdoor, with its expansive space, gives you the comfort of exercising as you wish without having to bump into the next person.

Avoid Unhealthy Competition

The outdoors gives you the freedom to exercise at your own pace. While at the gym, you can't help but glance at the next person, hoping they're not out running or out lifting you. If they are, you pick up the pace. You end up engaging in unhealthy competition by trying to match a person whose ability and goals are different from yours.

Get the Right Running Shoes for Your Feet Type
No matter which form of exercise you choose, you must carefully select your workout shoes. Your choice of shoes has a major impact on the results of your exercise routine. The first step in selecting the shoes is understanding the formation of your feet in relation to the arches. This basically refers to the ligament which runs between the heel and the ball at the base of your foot. The arch determines the manner in which the weight is distributed as you move.

The easiest way to test your arch is to step onto a brown paper bag with a wet foot, then categorize the imprint as follows:

Normal arch: The centre portion of the arch is just about halfway, with a distinct curve along the arch. This type of foot strikes just the right balance in absorbing and distributing your weight as you walk or run.

Flat Feet: The imprint is full, almost rectangular, without any significant curve at the centre. This means that the foot rolls inwards as you walk, bringing the entire surface into contact with the ground, a condition referred to as over-pronation.

High Arch: The curve at the middle is steep, and the imprint has almost nothing between the ball and the foot.

If you have a normal arch, you're lucky; the usual sports shoes will do just fine. Those with high or low arches have to be more careful, as these feet formations increase your risk of pains and injury. You should select customized shoes for each condition.

For flat feet, go for shoes that raised at the arch to keep the feet from rolling excessively and a thick cushioned sole for extra support. You can also find special inserts made for the above purposes that you slip into normal shoes to adapt for flat feet. These shoes tend to be straighter in shape and made from a rigid material to limit motion.

A high arch foot leaves empty space in the middle, and the shoe should compensate by cushioning this area to enable the foot to absorb pressure evenly. These shoes are more flexible as the foot itself is rigid. If you're on a tight budget, inserts will serve you well instead of going for customized shoes each time. You can buy the inserts from sport shoe shops or the pharmacy. Some of the inserts come in the form of socks which you wear with your shoes. If your arch is excessively high or low, consider consulting a doctor for a custom-made insert.

A rule of thumb when buying shoes is to do so in the afternoon, or basically after some physical activity when the feet have expanded to the maximum. If you try on shoes in the morning, they'll feel uncomfortably tight once you start moving around. Carry your running socks for the shopping trip and try them on together.

Workout shoes should fit snuggly. Let there be enough space to wiggle your toes without scraping them. Don't go for aesthetics, your favourite colour, or to match your running outfit while ignoring the basics like fit and comfort. Finally, change your shoes as often as necessary, as worn shoes increase the risk of injury.

Exercising Safely During Intermittent Fasting

Choose Simple Exercises

Your body is still adjusting to long periods without food and the reduced caloric intake. Go for simple exercises to avoid exerting undue strain and causing adrenal fatigue. Regulated exercise should leave you more energetic, not miserably worn out. You can start with yoga, then proceed to walk, then jog, eventually going for runs as your body allows. Swimming is also a great option as it takes the weight of the body off the joints.

Hydrate

Have your bottle of water close. When working out, you lose even more water due to sweating, and you need to periodically replenish by drinking more water. Hydrating will also help you fight hunger pangs if you're exercising while fasting. Beware of energy/sports drink; they could contain calories and should only be taken if you're exercising in the eating phase.

Control Intensity and Duration

If you've not been exercising much, and especially if you're overweight, you should choose low impact exercises that exert minimal pressure on the body. Of key importance here is joint health. Having to carry all your weight through the workout is no mean feat. If you're accustomed to a sedentary lifestyle where you spend most of the time sitting at your desk, you're likely to have knee and ankle pains after a workout session. Choose less intense workouts, and even then, keep the duration relatively short.

Consider your Fasting Plan

Longer fasting sessions should be accompanied by lighter workout sessions and vice versa. If you're fasting for an entire 24 hours, include only minimal impact exercises. If on a 12 hour fast, you can go for something more intense. Working out in the fed state will also allow you more vigour compared to the fasting state.

Listen to your Body

Do not exercise through joint pain, headaches, dizziness or extremely low energy. Such strain will not only compromise the effectiveness of your fast but could also leave you nursing an injury. Your body is a rather accurate gauge; it knows when it's had enough. If it's telling you to go slow, you should.

Chapter 14: Overcoming down moments in IF

When it comes to one's ultimate health and desire to achieve the targets, controlling appetite and keeping healthy food is important. Intermittent fasting will help you accomplish this, but although certain individuals can fast with very little problem for long stretches, some people can find it a bit more challenging, particularly when they first start.

There are many women who have successfully started doing intermittent fasting. The first thing you need to know is that you will have to eat. Skip breakfast and then eat a small lunch, followed by another small lunch, and then a very large dinner. The reasoning is that you won't be hungry because you haven't had breakfast, and all your hormones shake-up will make you not want to eat. You will have to make sure that you eat healthy foods. Healthy food is one that is low in sugar, butter, oil, salt and anything else that is high in fat. You can not eat greasy, high sugar lunch if you are going to skip breakfast and still be able to fast for 16 more hours. Eat lean protein, such as chicken and fish. Those that have the highest protein content include turkey breast and other lean cuts of meat. Eating vegetables with your meal is always a good idea. It's best to eat vegetables like lettuce, spinach, and broccoli that are low in sugar.

The size of your lunch will depend on the size of your dinner. Don't eat too much, or you will have problems with digestion. If you can't stand the hunger, choose a night snack; a few nuts, a piece of high-protein cheese such as cheddar, or a handful of unsalted pretzels. Skip the sweets and chocolate. They are not a good idea if you plan to fast until dinner. Before dinner, you can drink non-caffeinated tea or water or other clear fluids. Caffeine is a stimulant and will make it harder to fast.

A good way to count your calories when you eat is to use the calorie calculator. This will help you make sure that you aren't overeating. Overeating will give you more calories than you need. You need to make sure that you stay under the recommended calories for your age and gender.

Although intermittent fasting can be very challenging, you can gradually increase the amount of time you fast. Fasting will give your body an opportunity to use its energy in other ways. When you fast, your body can use its energy to make the cells stronger. When you give your body this time and focus, it will have an opportunity to rest and recuperate during the fasting time. If you don't have a hard time with this practice, there are signs that you are becoming an expert at it. These signs include relaxed skin, no hunger pangs, and weight loss. Don't ever lose sight of why you are trying it in the first place. In the beginning, it can seem like an all-day event. You'll need to find a balance. You will want to do it for the right reasons, so don't try to push yourself too hard. It's usually just 2-4 days per week. If you work, you can start to have your fast on a few mornings in the week. You will need to find a balance of your schedule. Some of the tips that will help you remember are to try and fit the fast into your life and try and mind the window of time you have to fast. If you're planning to fast most days, you'll need to do it before work. This will cut down the chance of cravings, and you'll get used to it. Suppose you're having problems with hunger, only fast for the small window of time. Do not allow yourself to get hungry. This will help you to stick to the plan.

Remember to drink a large cup of water with your meal; a few hours later, you should also be able to drink a cup of water to stay hydrated before your next meal. If you find that you can't stop, you may be overdoing it. Try eating very small amounts with water throughout the day, rather than large meals. This will help you to maintain your fasting for longer. Keep in mind that this isn't something to do with losing weight. Stay as healthy as you can.

This method of fasting is a good way to keep your body healthy and strong, and it will make you feel better in every way. On a daily basis, doing 15 or 20 minutes of intermittent fasting will not cause any harm. If you can start this practice, you will be amazed at the difference in your health, weight, and outlook on life.

There is a set of ideas to help you out that one can use to get the best results and make the ride a little smoother.

Start the Fast After Dinner

One of the best advice one can offer is when you do regular or weekly fasting is to begin the fast after dinner. Using this ensures you're going to be sleeping for a good portion of the fasting time. Especially when using a daily fasting method like 16:8

Eat More Satisfying Meals

The type of food one consume affects their willingness to both the urge to complete the fast and what you crave to eat after the fast. Too much salty and sugary foods with making you hungrier rather than consume meals that are homey satisfying and will help you lose weight

• Morning eggs or oats porridge

• A healthy lunch of chicken breast, baked sweet potato, and veggies.

• After the workout, drink a protein milkshake.

• Then you end the day in the evening with an equally impressive dinner.

Control Your Appetite

Without question, while fasting, hunger pangs can set in from start to end. The trick as this occurs is to curb your appetite, and with Zero-calorie beverages that help provide satiety and hold hunger at bay before it's time to break the fast, the perfect way to do this is. Examples of food to consume are

• Sparkling water

• Water

• Black tea

• Black coffee

• Green tea

• Herbal teas and other zero-calorie unsweetened drinks

Stay Busy

Boredom is the main threat. It is the invisible assassin who, bit by bit, creeps in to ruin the progress, breaking you down steadily and dragging you downwards. For a second, think about it. How often boredom has caused you to consume more than you can, intend to, or even know that you are. Hence try to plan your day.

Stick to A Routine

Start and break your fast each day at regular times. You are consuming a diet weekly where you finish similar items per day—meal prepping in advance. Making a plan allows things easier to adhere to the IF schedule, so you eliminate the uncertainty and second-guessing the process until you learn what works for you and commit to it every day. Follow-through is what one has to do.

Give Yourself Time to Adjust

When one first starts intermittent fasting, odds are you're going to mess up a couple of times; this is both OK and natural. It's just normal to have hunger pangs. This doesn't mean that you have to give up or that it's not going to be effective for you. Alternatively, it's a chance to learn, to ask whether or how you messed up, and take action to deter it from occurring again.

Enjoy Yourself

Let yourself enjoy the process. No one starts at the pro level, so you should go out with your friends and attend those birthday parties as well.

Chapter 15: Manage menopause

Here are five remedies for five symptoms that are common among women in their forties and fifties. (Remember, any questions you have should always be discussed with your healthcare provider first.) Other medications or potentially adverse side effects can be available. You should decide the choices are better for you as a couple.)

1. Mood Changes

Hormone fluctuations during perimenopause can leave some women feeling out of control. Increased irritability, anxiety, exhaustion, and depressed moods are common complaints. Relaxation and stress-reduction strategies, such as deep-breathing exercises and massage, as well as a healthy lifestyle (including good diet and physical exercise) and fun, self-nurturing activities, can all be beneficial. Some people use over-the-counter remedies like St. John's wort or vitamin B6 to alleviate menopause symptoms.

Discussing your mood problems with your doctor will help you figure out what's causing them, check for serious depression, and decide on the best course of action. Prescription antidepressant drugs can be prescribed for depression to remedy a chemical imbalance. While it takes many weeks to feel the full effect of one of these treatments, several women report significant improvements with very few side effects. Hot flashes have been shown to be treated by certain antidepressants. When antidepressant treatment is combined with counselling or psychotherapy, it is most effective.

2. Urinary Incontinence
Although urinary incontinence is described as the involuntary loss of urine over time, most women would describe it as an unfortunate, unexpected, and unwanted nuisance. Fortunately, there are non-surgical and

nonmedication methods for treating different types of incontinence. To keep urine filtered (clear and pale yellow), drink plenty of water and avoid foods or drinks rich in acid or caffeine, which can irritate the bladder lining. Grapefruit, bananas, tomatoes, coffee, and caffeine-containing soft drinks are among them. To strengthen the pelvic floor muscles and reduce incontinence episodes, try Kegel exercises.

3. Sweats at Night

Try these various ways to stay calm while sleeping to get relief from night sweats (hot flashes that occur during sleep):

- Dress in light nightclothes.
- Use layered bedding that can easily be removed during the night.
- Or, try wicking materials for both.
- Cool down with an electric fan.
- Sip cool water throughout the night

Keep a frozen cold pack under your pillow and flip it over often, so your head is always resting on a cool surface, or place a cold pack on your feet.

4. Having a Hard Time Falling Asleep

Establish a consistent sleep schedule and routine:

- Even on weekends, get up and go to bed at the same times every day.
- Before going to bed, unwind and relax by reading a book, listening to music, or taking a long bath.
- Tryptophan is found in milk and peanuts, and it helps the body relax.
- A cup of chamomile tea could also help.
- Maintain a comfortable amount of light, noise, and temperature in your bedroom — dark, quiet, and cool are conducive to sleep.

- Use the bedroom for sleeping and sex.
- Avoid caffeine and alcohol.

5. Sexual Dissatisfaction

Menopause causes changes in sexual function by reducing ovarian hormone output, which can cause vaginal dryness and a decline in sexual function. To combat these changes, try the following:

Vaginal lubricants: These drugs, which are available without a prescription, reduce pressure and make intercourse easier when the vagina is dry. Since oil-based products like Vaseline can irritate the skin, only water-soluble products should be used. Just use vaginal products; avoid hand creams and lotions that contain alcohol or perfumes, as well as warming/tingling and flavoured lubricants that may irritate sensitive tissue. (Astroglide, Moist Again, and Silk-E are some of the vaginal lubricants available.)

Vaginal moisturizers: These items, which are often available without a prescription, help people with moderate vaginal atrophy preserve or increase vaginal moisture (when tissues of the vulva and the lining of the vagina become thin, dry, less elastic, and less lubricated as a result of estrogen loss). They also keep the pH of the vaginal environment low, ensuring a safe vaginal environment. Replens and K-Y Long-lasting Vaginal Moisturizer are two examples.) These drugs are more long-lasting than vaginal lubricants and can be used on a regular basis.

Last but not least, women can maintain vaginal health by engaging in painless sexual activity on a regular basis, which increases blood flow to the genital region.

Menopause Natural Treatments That Actually Work

Women who don't want to use hormone therapy to relieve their menopause symptoms have a number of options that can be very successful. For memory issues, weight gain, high cholesterol, and vaginal symptoms, here are some natural lifestyle tips.

Natural Remedies: A Word of Caution

Always keep in mind that normally does not imply risk-free. Many herbal, fruit and dietary supplements may interfere with prescription drugs or worsen chronic medical conditions. Natural methods are not without risk, and the more you know, the better equipped you will be to select therapies that will keep you healthy and secure.

Check with your medical professional before choosing to use alternative and complementary treatments for your menopause symptoms, and read up on any potential side effects and cautions for any remedy you're considering.

Memory Problems

It's aggravating to try to remember a word or name that's on the tip of your tongue, but you can't get it out. As you prepare to leave the house, forgetting where you put your car keys or where you put your glasses will drive you insane. Does this ring a bell? When they approach perimenopause, many women begin to notice memory problems. There are things you can do to keep your memory when you grow older, even though it's just the normal ageing process.

Green tea consumption has been linked to a variety of health benefits, including the enhancement of the immune system and the prevention of cancer. Green tea is now being linked to preventing memory-damaging enzyme activity in studies. It has a small number of side effects and is widely available.

A sufficient amount of sleep is needed for your brain to process memory tasks. Both short and longer naps seem to help memory work, according to research. If you can't get a cat nap during the day, make sure you get enough overnight sleep to avoid memory issues.

Control of stress: Stress is a big memory sapper. Pay attention to your stress level, whether you're having trouble focusing or recalling everyday things. Even short-term stress has been shown to affect learning and memory, according to research. Divorce, illness, raising children, and elderly parents are only a few of the issues that can arise during the menopause process. It is a survival skill to take care of yourself and reduce tension in your life. Memory issues may be an early warning sign that the stress level is rising.

Weight Gain

For women over 50, weight gain is often a source of irritation. The exact mechanism by which estrogen affects metabolism is unknown. What is obvious, however, is that many women who have never struggled to maintain a healthy weight before menopause continue to do so during and after the menopause era. Although there are no validated herbal weight loss remedies, there are lifestyle and dietary improvements that can help you naturally reduce your weight gain.

Stress management: Stress, especially the production of the stress hormone cortisol, may impair your body's ability to maintain a healthy weight.

It would be easier for your body to regulate calories and fat metabolism if you keep cortisol levels down.

Diet must-haves include: The menopause process is an excellent opportunity to review your diet and make lifestyle adjustments that will benefit you for the rest of your life. You should amend your thinking to include a good menopause diet that will set the stage for a balanced postmenopause as your metabolism slows and you begin to treat calories differently.

Everyone agrees that exercise is beneficial to one's health. However, when you approach menopause, it becomes an essential part of the overall health strategy. Weight loss, of course, necessitates increased physical activity. Exercise, on the other hand, is an all-purpose solution to menopause wellbeing since it improves memory, mood, and bone health. Exercise is the only thing that can help you control your weight to its full potential.

Sleep: You would think that getting enough sleep would sabotage your weight loss efforts, but the opposite is true. When you don't get enough sleep, it makes you want to eat more and causes your body to store fat around your midsection. A good night's sleep helps the body reset and recover from the pressures of the day. If you get enough sleep, the body can function more effectively in any way.

Cholesterol levels are high.

As estrogen levels drop during menopause, your cholesterol levels will rise. Women are soon at the same risk as men for heart disease. You can lower cholesterol levels in a number of natural ways.

Soy and red clover: Soy protein has been shown to lower "bad" (LDL) cholesterol and lower total cholesterol levels. Red clover appears to increase "good" (HDL) cholesterol while lowering triglycerides. It's possible that these plant estrogens step in to protect your heart when your own estrogen levels drop.

Whole grain oats: Including whole grain oats in your diet will reduce total and LDL cholesterol levels, lowering cardiac risk.

Melatonin: Melatonin can help raise HDL cholesterol levels without increasing overall cholesterol levels, in addition to assisting with sleep. This may be beneficial for women who have a higher risk of heart disease. If you're taking melatonin for sleep, you might notice that it lowers your cholesterol as a side effect.

Symptoms of the Vaginal Canal

Two concerns that women may have difficulty getting to their doctors are the loss of satisfaction during sexual intercourse and the beginning of urine leakage. There are a few things you can do if you're getting vaginal symptoms as you approach menopause:

Wild yam cream: Creams made from wild yam contain a phytoestrogen that, like other estrogen creams, can help relieve symptoms locally.

Vitamin E and flaxseed oil: Whether taken orally or applied directly to the vagina, the combination of vitamin E and flaxseed oil may provide some relief from vaginal and urinary symptoms. Women usually take them as oral supplements, but creams containing them may also be applied directly to the vaginal region.

Kegel exercises can help to strengthen the pelvic floor muscles and enhance intercourse sensation while also reducing urinary incontinence.

You can see results in 2 to 4 weeks if you do them many times a day. Vaginal moisturizers and lubricants: Vaginal moisturizers operate for many days to make the vagina more elastic, and vaginal lubricants help minimize friction and pain throughout intercourse. Water-based products are less likely to cause an allergic reaction and are widely available in pharmacies.

How To Lose Weight During Menopause

Weight gain is common among women going through the menopausal process. Many that want to lose this weight can find it more difficult than normal to do so, and keeping it off can be difficult.

Part of the reason for weight gain before and after menopause is a decrease in estrogen levels.

Weight gain can also be caused by insufficient sleep and age-related changes in metabolism and muscle tone. The abdomen is where much of the weight accumulates.

While losing weight during menopause can be more difficult, many people find that there are a variety of methods that work.

· Weight gain during menopause

- After a period of 12 months without a menstrual cycle, women hit menopause.
- People can gain body fat and find it difficult to lose weight during menopause and perimenopause (the period leading up to menopause).

For the following factors, menopause is related to a rise in body fat:

Estrogen levels dropping

- Weight gain is caused by changes in estrogen levels.
- In females, estrogen is one of the most important sex hormones.

It's involved in:

- physical features of a sex maintaining bone health controlling
- cholesterol levels regulating the menstrual cycle
- Estrogen levels drop dramatically during menopause.

Low estrogen levels during menopause do not cause weight gain directly, but they can increase overall body fat and abdominal fat. Excess weight in middle age is linked to heart disease and type 2 diabetes, according to doctors.

Hormone replacement therapy can help to reduce abdominal fat gain.

Processes of the natural ageing

Regular ageing processes and lifestyle patterns are also related to weight gain during menopause.

People appear to become less physically involved as they get older. Their metabolism slows down naturally as well. These factors result in a loss of muscle mass and an increase in body fat.

Poor Sleep

Doctors also connect menopause to sleep problems, which can be caused by hot flashes or night sweats. Sleep deprivation has been linked to weight gain in animals.

The following are some weight-loss techniques for women going through menopause.

1. Increasing activity

Daily exercise is a great way to lose weight and improve your overall health.

Many people's muscle tone deteriorates as they age, and this deterioration can lead to a rise in body fat. Exercise is an essential part of maintaining muscle mass and preventing age-related muscle loss.
Aerobic activity has been shown in studies to help women lose weight after menopause. Resistance training three days a week can increase lean body

mass and minimize body fat in postmenopausal women, according to another report.

According to the Physical Activity Guidelines for Americans, people should strive for at least 150 minutes of aerobic activity per week and two or three days of muscle-strengthening activities per week.

Body fat will be reduced, and muscle will be built by a combination of aerobic exercise and resistance training.

If an individual isn't already involved, gradually increasing their activity levels can be easier. The following are some easy ways to incorporate more exercise into your day:

doing yard work, such as gardening, walking a puppy, taking the stairs instead of the elevator, standing up to take phone calls going for a walk, or getting another form of exercise at lunchtime.

2. Consuming nutrient-dense foods

People must eat fewer calories than they expend in order to lose weight. Dietary improvements are an essential part of losing weight.

All meals and snacks should be built around nutritious, nutrient-dense foods. Colourful fruits and vegetables, whole grains, and lean protein sources can all be included in a person's diet.

According to a 2016 study, this diet can help with heart disease risk factors, including blood pressure and lipid levels, as well as weight loss.

People should make it a point to eat at least once a day:
a wide range of fruits and vegetables lean proteins such as beans, fish, and chicken whole grains in bread and cereals

Olive oil and avocados are good sources of healthy fats, as are legumes.

Processed foods, as well as those rich in trans or saturated fats, should be avoided. Here are a few examples:

- white bread pastries, such as cakes, cookies, and doughnuts
- processed meats with a lot of added oils or sugar, such as hot dogs
- or bologna
- Reduced intake of sweetened beverages, such as sodas and juices, can also benefit. Sugar-sweetened drinks have high-calorie content.

A dietician or nutritionist may assist you in developing a healthy eating plan and keeping track of your progress.

3. Setting sleep as a top priority

It's important to get enough good sleep to maintain a healthy weight and overall health. Sleep deprivation can lead to weight gain.

- Sleep disruptions have been related to ageing and metabolic disruption during menopause in studies. Changes in sleep quality and circadian rhythms may have an effect on: hormones that control
- hunger
- energy expenditure body fat composition
- Symptoms like hot flashes and night sweats can also make it difficult to sleep.

Menopause-related weight gain can be reduced by focusing on having enough restful sleep.

4. Considering complementary and alternative treatments

Overall, there hasn't been a lot of well-conducted, definitive research into whether alternative medicine can help with menopause symptoms.

Although these treatments are unlikely to result in substantial weight loss, they can aid in the relief of certain symptoms and the reduction of stress.

The following are some examples of complementary and alternative therapies:

- Yoga Hypnosis
- herbal remedies
- and meditation
- Restaurant portion sizes have risen over time, and people are eating out more, making it difficult to determine how much food a person requires per meal and per day.

Understanding the regular serving sizes of certain popular foods will aid in determining how much to include in a meal. For instance, here are some typical servings:

12 cup cooked fruit – one small piece milk or yoghurt – bread – 1 slice rice and pasta – 12 cups cooked fruit – 1 cup cheese – 2 ounces meat or fish (the size of a domino) – 2 to 3 ounces meat or fish (the size of a deck of cards)

The following suggestions will assist people in controlling their portion sizes:

- Instead of eating snacks straight from the bag, measure them out.
- Instead of sitting in front of the tv, eat at a table.
- When dining out, order fewer appetizers and less bread.
- To weigh portions at home, use a kitchen scale and measuring cups.

8. Make preparations ahead of time

In a pinch, meal preparation and keeping healthy foods on hand will make it less likely for a person to select unhealthy foods.

Stock the kitchen with nutritious foods for fast meals, and prepare ahead of time to avoid impulsive, mindless eating. To avoid visits to the vending machine, bring healthy snacks with you.

9. Enlisting the assistance of friends and family

Having a love of family and friends is crucial when it comes to losing weight. For example, having a workout buddy can help people stay motivated to exercise.

Some people use social media to monitor their success, which may help with accountability.

10. Making lifestyle improvements

The trick to losing weight, in the long run, is to maintain healthy habits.

Short-term weight loss is more likely with fad diets, while long-term results are more likely with healthy practices such as cooking routines and daily exercise.

Chapter 16: Days meal plan

Intermittent fasting is simply you eating all your meals and snacks for the day in a short and specific window of time, say between noon and 8.p.m. So, if you're new to intermittent fasting and are wondering how to go about it, here are some meal plans with recipes to aid you in your journey to perfect health.

This meal plan can be repeated as often as you want it.

Day 1

Brunch

Eggs, Scrambled with Sweet Potato

Prep & Cooking time: 25 minutes

Servings: 1

Ingredients

- 1   (8-oz) sweet potato, diced
- ½ cup chopped onion
- 2   teaspoons (tsp.) chopped rosemary
- Salt
- Pepper
- 4 large eggs
- Four large egg whites
- 2 tablespoons (tbsp.) of chopped chive

Direction

1. Heat the oven beforehand to 425°F. Toss the sweet potato, onion, rosemary, salt, and pepper on a baking sheet. Roast until tender for 20 minutes after spraying with cooking spray.
2. In a medium-sized bowl, whisk together the eggs, egg white, adding a pinch of pepper and salt to it. With the cooking spray, spritz the pan and scramble the eggs for about 5 minutes on the medium.
3. Have chopped chives sprinkled on it and then serve with the potatoes.

Nutritional value per serving: Calorie content: 571, 44 g protein, 52 g carbs (9 g fibre), 20 g fat

Dinner

Turkey Tacos

Prep & Cooking time: 25 minutes

Servings: 4

Ingredients

- 2 tsp. of oil
- 1 small red onion, chopped
- 1 clove garlic, finely chopped
- 1 lb. extra-lean ground turkey
- 1 tbsp sodium-free taco seasoning
- 8 whole-grain corn tortillas, warmed
- ¼ cup sour cream
- ½ cup shredded Mexican cheese
- 1 avocado, sliced
- Salsa, for serving
- 1 cup chopped lettuce

Directions

1. On a high medium, heat the oil using a large pan. Stir till it is tender. Add the onions and cook for about 5-6 minutes. Add the garlic and cook for about a minute. The turkey should be added, breaking with a spoon, and cook for 5 minutes until nearly brown. Put the taco seasoning and one cup of water. For 7 minutes, simmer until reduced to slightly more than half.
2. With turkey, fill up the tortillas topping them with cheese, sour cream, avocado, lettuce, and salsa.

Nutritional value per serving: Calorie content: 472, 28 g protein, 30 g carbs (6 g fibre), 27 g fat

Day 2 Brunch

Greek Chickpea Waffles

Prep & Cooking time: 30 minutes

Servings: 2

Ingredients for making

- ¾ cup of chickpea flour
- ½ tsp. of baking soda
- ½ tsp. of salt
- ¾ cup of plain Greek yoghurt (2%)
- 6 eggs (large ones)
- Tomatoes, scallion, cucumbers, olive oil, lemon juice, yoghurt, and parsley for serving (optional) • Salt and pepper **Directions**

1. Heat the oven beforehand to 200°F. Over a rimmed baking sheet, set a wire rack over it and place it in the oven, per direction, heat waffle iron.
2. Whisk together in a large bowl the flour, baking soda, and salt. While in a small bowl, whisk the egg and yoghurt together. Mix the wet ingredients into the dry ingredients.
3. With a nonstick cooking spray, lightly coat the waffle iron. Drop-in batches ¼ to ½ cup batter into each section of the iron. For about 4 to 5 minutes, cook till it becomes golden brown. Open up the oven and put the waffles in there to keep them warm. Keep this process going on and on with the remaining batter.
4.
5. Mix in the savoury tomato or a drizzle of warm nut butter and berries, and then you can serve the waffles.

Nutritional value per serving: Calorie content: 412, 35 g protein, 24 g carbs (4 g fibre), 18 g fat

Dinner

Healthy Spaghetti Bolognese

Prep & Cooking time: 1 hour and 30 minutes

Servings: 4

Ingredients

- 1 large spaghetti squash
- 3 tbsp. olive oil
- ½ tsp. garlic powder
- Kosher salt and pepper
- 1 small onion, finely chopped
- 1¼ lb. ground turkey
- 4 cloves garlic, finely chopped
- 8 oz. small cremini mushrooms, sliced
- 3 cups fresh diced tomatoes (or two 15-oz cans)
- 1 (8-oz.) can low-sodium, no-sugar-added tomato
- sauce Fresh chopped basil **Direction**

1. First and foremost, the oven should be heated to 400°F. Likewise, cut the spaghetti in half, squash, and discard the seed with 1/2 tbsp. Oil, rub each half and season with ¼ tsp: each salt, pepper, and garlic powder. Within 55 to 40 minutes, roast till tender placing them skinside up on a rimmed baking sheet. Allow cooling for about 10 minutes.

2. For the time being, heat the remaining 2 tbsp oil on a large pan on a medium. At the same time, it is adding the onions, season with pepper and ¼ tsp. Each of salt. Occasionally stirring, cook till it becomes tender for 360 seconds. Add the turkey and cook, breaking it up into smaller pieces with a spoon for 6 to 7 minutes till it becomes brown. In garlic, stir and cook for a minute.

3. Partition the pan pushing the turkey mixture to one side while placing the mushrooms at the other. In 5 minutes, cook, occasionally stirring till the mushrooms are tender. Mix into the turkey. Add your tomato sauce and tomatoes simmering for at least 10 minutes.

4. Scoop up the squash and transfer to plates while the sauce is simmering. If desired, spoon the turkey Bolognese over the top and sprinkle with basil.

Nutritional value per serving: Calorie content: 450, 32 g protein, 31 g carbs (6 g fibre), 23 g fat

Day 3 Brunch

PB&J Overnight Oats

Prep & Cooking time: 5 minutes (and 8 hours refrigeration)

Servings: 1

Ingredients

- ¼ cup quick-cooking rolled oats
- ½ cup 2 per cent milk
- 3 tbsp. creamy peanut butter
- ¼ cup mashed raspberries
- 3 tbsp. whole raspberries

Directions

1. Combine in a medium bowl oat, milk, peanut butter, and mashed raspberries. Stir till it becomes smooth. Cover the content and refrigerate through the night. In the morning, uncover, spray whole raspberries as a topping.

Nutritional value per serving: Calorie content: 455, 20 g protein, 36 g carbs (9 g fibre), 28 g fat

Dinner

Chicken with Fried Cauliflower Rice

Prep & Cooking time: 35 minutes

Servings: 4

Ingredients for making

- 2 tbsp. of grapeseed oil
- 1   ¼ lb. chicken breast without bones or skin (pounded to eventhickness) 4 beaten large eggs
- 2   finely chopped red bell peppers
-

- 2 small carrots, finely chopped
- 1 finely chopped onions
- 2 finely chopped cloves of garlic
- 4 finely chopped scallions, plus more for serving
- ½ cup frozen peas, thawed
- 4 cups cauliflower "rice."
- 2 tbsp. low-sodium soy sauce
- 2 tsp. rice vinegar
- Kosher salt and pepper

Directions

1. In a large deep pan, heat 1tbsp of oil over medium-high heat. Add the chicken and for 3 to 4 minutes, cook till it becomes golden brown per side. The chicken should be transferred to a chopping board and be left for 6 minutes before slicing. Add the remaining 1tbsp of oil to the frying pan. Add the eggs and scramble till it is set. 1 to 2 minutes later, transfer it to a bowl.
2. Add the bell pepper, carrot, and onion to the frying pan and cook, often stirring, till it becomes tender for 4 to 5 minutes—Cook for a minute stirring in the garlic. Toss with peas and scallions.
3. Add the soy sauce, cauliflower, rice vinegar, salt, and pepper, and toss to combine. Without stirring, let the cauliflower sit till it's beginning to turn brown for 2 to 3 minutes. Toss with egg and sliced chicken.

Nutritional value per serving: Calorie content: 427, 45 g protein, 25 g carbs (7 g fibre), 16 g fat

Day 4 Brunch

Turmeric Tofu Scramble

Prep & Cooking time: 15 minutes

Servings: 1

Required ingredients

- 1 portobello mushroom
- 3 to 4 cherry tomatoes
- 1 tbsp. of olive oil (and more for brushing)
- Salt and pepper
- ½ block (14-oz) firm tofu
- ¼ tsp. ground turmeric
- Pinch garlic powder
- ½ avocado, thinly sliced

Directions

1. Heat the oven to 400°F. Place the mushroom and tomatoes on a baking sheet brushing them with oil. Season with pepper and salt. Roast for 10 minutes till it becomes tender.
2. During the time, combine the tofu, turmeric, garlic powder, and a pinch of salt in a medium bowl. Then mash with a fork. Over medium heat, heat up a tbsp of olive oil in a large frying pan. Add the tofu mixture and cook for about 3 minutes, occasionally stirring till firm and egg-like.
3. Serve the tofu with the mushroom, avocado, and tomatoes on a plate.

Nutritional value per serving: Calorie content: 431, 21 g protein, 17 g carbs (8 g fibre), 33 g fat

Dinner

Sheet Pan Steak

Prep & Cooking time: 50 minutes
Servings: 4

Required ingredients

- 1 lb. small cremini mushrooms, trimmed and halved
- 1 ¼ lb. bunch broccolini, trimmed and cut into 2-in. lengths
- 4 finely chopped cloves of garlic
- 3 tbsp. of olive oil
- ¼ tsp. of red pepper flakes
- Kosher salt and pepper
- 2 1-inch thick New York strip steaks (about 1½ lb total), trimmed of excess fat
- 1 15-oz. can low-sodium cannellini beans, rinsed **Directions**

1. Heat up the oven to 450°F. Mix in the mushrooms, broccolini, garlic, oil, red pepper flakes, and ¼ tsp. Each salt and pepper on a large, rimmed baking sheet. Roast for 15 minutes, place the baking sheet inside the oven.
2. Make room for the steak by pushing the mixture to the end of the pan. At the centre of the pan, Place the steak you have seasoned with ¼ tsp. of salt and pepper. For a medium-rare per side, roast the steak to your desired taste for 5 to 7 minutes. Transfer the steak to a chopping board. Let it cool for 5 minutes before slicing it.
3. To the baking sheet, add the beans and toss to combine them. Roast until it is thoroughly heated for 3 minutes, then serve vegetables and the beans with meat.

Nutritional value per serving: Calorie content: 464, 42 g protein, 26 g carbs (8 g fibre), 22 g fat

Day 5 Brunch

Avocado Ricotta Power Toast

Prep & Cooking time: 5 minutes

Servings: 1

Ingredients

- 1   slice whole-grain bread
- ¼ ripe avocado smashed
- 2   tbsp. ricotta
- Pinch crushed red pepper flakes
- Pinch flaky sea salt

Directions

1. The bread should be toasted. Top with crushed red pepper flakes, avocado, sea salt, and ricotta. Eat it with boiled or scrambled eggs with fruit or yoghurt.

Nutritional value per serving: Calorie content: 288, 10 g protein, 29 g carbs (10 g fibre), 17 g fat

Dinner

Pork Tenderloin with Butternut Squash and Brussels Sprouts

Prep & Cooking time: 50 minutes

Servings: 4

Ingredients

- 1¾ lb. pork tenderloin, trimmed
- Salt
- Pepper
- 3 tbsp. canola oil
- 2 sprigs of fresh thyme
- 2 garlic cloves, peeled
- 4 cups Brussels sprouts, trimmed and halved
- 4 cups diced butternut squash

Directions

1. The oven should be heated first to 400°F. Use salt and pepper to season the tenderloin all over. Over medium-high, heat 1 tbsp. Of the oil on a large cast-iron pan. Add tenderloin as soon as the oil

shimmers and sear for 8 to 12 minutes till it becomes golden brown on all sides. Then transfer to a plate.

2. Add the remaining 2 tbsp. Of oil with thyme, garlic to the pan and cook till aromatic for a minute.
3. Take a big pinch out of the salt and pepper, add the Brussels sprouts, the butternut squash to it. In 4 to 6 minutes, cook, occasionally stirring till the vegetables becomes a bit brown.
4. Place the tenderloin on top of the vegetables and put everything inside the oven. For 15 to 20 minutes, roast till the vegetables become tender, and on the meat, the thermometer is registered 140°F.
5. Take the pan out of the oven, cautiously, with oven mitts. Let the tenderloin cool off for 5 minutes before slicing and serving with vegetables. To serve as a side, toss greens with balsamic vinaigrette to it.

Nutritional value per serving: Calorie content: 401, 44 g protein, 25 g carbs (6 g fibre), 15 g fat

Day 6 Brunch

Turkish Egg Breakfast

Prep & Cooking time: 13 minutes

Servings: 2

Ingredients

- 2 tbsp. olive oil
- ¾ cup diced red bell pepper
- ¾ cup diced eggplant
- Pinch each of salt and pepper
- 5 large eggs, lightly beaten
- ¼ tsp. paprika
- Chopped cilantro to taste
- 2 dollops plain yoghurt
- 1 whole-wheat pita

Directions

1. On a medium-high, heat the olive oil in a large nonstick pan. Add salt, pepper, eggplant, and bell pepper. For 7 minutes, Sauté till it is softened. Stir the paprika, egg with more pepper and salt to taste. Continue stirring till the eggs become beat.
2. Sprinkle chopped cilantro on it and serve with pita and a dollop of yoghurt.

Nutritional value per serving: Calorie content: 469, 25 g protein, 26 g carbs (4 g fibre), 29 g fat

Dinner

Wild Cajun Spiced Salmon

Prep & Cooking time: 30 minutes

Servings: 4

Required ingredients

- 1½ lb. wild Alaskan salmon fillet
- Sodium-free taco seasoning
- ½ head (about 1 lb) of cauliflower cut into florets
- 1 head (about 1 lb) of broccoli cut into florets
- 3   tbsp. of olive oil
- ½ tsp. of garlic powder
- 4   diced tomatoes, medium size

Directions

1. First, heat the oven to 375 °F. In the baking dish, place the salmon. With ½ cup water in a small dish, mix the taco seasoning. Pour this mixture over to the salmon, and for 12 to 15 minutes, bake till it becomes opaque throughout.
2.
3. For the time being, pulse the cauliflower and broccoli until finely chopped and "riced" in a food processor.
4. Over medium heat, pour in the oil in a large frying pan to heat up. The cauliflower and broccoli should be added sprinkle with garlic powder. Cook for five to about six minutes till it becomes tender.

5. The salmon can be served on top of rice, with tomatoes on top.

Nutritional value per serving: Calorie content: 408, 42 g protein, 9 g carbs (3 g fibre), 23 g fat

Day 7

Brunch

Almond Apple Spice Muffins

Prep & Cooking time: 15 minutes | Servings: 5

Ingredients

- ½ stick butter
- 2 cups almond meal
- 4 scoops of vanilla protein powder
- 4 large eggs
- 1 cup unsweetened applesauce
- 1 tbsp. cinnamon
- 1 tsp. allspice
- 1 tsp. cloves
- 2 tsp. baking powder**Directions**

1. First, heat the oven to 350°F. Over low heat, melt the butter in the microwave in a small microwave-safe bowl for about 30 seconds.
2. Mix thoroughly in a large bowl all the remaining ingredients with the melted butter. Using nonstick cooking spray or use cupcake liners, spray 2 muffin tins.
3.
4. Get muffin tins in which you pour the mixture; make sure not to fill it to the brim (about ¾ full). This should make 10 muffins.
5. In the one tray, you have placed in the oven, bake for 12 minutes. Endeavour not to over-bake so as not to make the muffin too dry. When you're done with the first tray, remove it from the oven and do likewise to the other muffin tins.

Nutritional value per serving: Calorie content: 484, 40 g protein, 16 g carbs (5 g fibre), 31 g fat

Dinner

Pork Chops with Bloody Mary Tomato Salad
Prep & Cooking time: 25 minutes

Servings: 4

Required ingredients

- 2 tbsp. of olive oil
- 2 tbsp. of red wine vinegar
- 2 tsp. of Worcestershire sauce
- 2 tsp. of squeezed dry prepared horseradish
- ½ tsp. of Tabasco
- ½ tsp. of celery seeds Kosher salt
- 1   pint of halved cherry tomatoes
- 2   very thinly sliced celery stalks
- ½ thinly sliced small red onion
- 4 (1 in. thick, about 2¼ lb total) small bone-in pork chops
- Pepper
- ¼ cup finely chopped flat-leaf parsley
- 1 small head green-leaf lettuce, leaves torn

Directions

1. The grill should be heated to medium-high. Mix in the oil, vinegar, Worcestershire sauce, horseradish, Tabasco, celery seeds, and ¼ tsp. of salt in a large bowl. With the addition of tomatoes, celery, and onion.
2. The Pork chops should be seasoned with ½ tsp. each salt and pepper
3. Grill it till it becomes golden brown and cook each side for 5 to 7 minutes.
4. The parsley should be folded into the tomatoes and serve over pork and greens. Eat it with mashed potatoes or cauliflower.

Nutritional value per serving: Calorie content: 400, 39 g protein, 8 g carbs (3 g fibre), 23 g fat

Chapter 17: Recipes

IF sides and snack recipes (at least 10)

Brussels sprouts chips

Prep & Cooking Time: 15-20 mins   Servings: 4

Ingredients:

- 1 lb. Brussels sprouts washed and dried, ends trimmed
- 1   tsp salt
- 2   tbsps extra virgin olive oil
- Smoked paprika, for serving

Directions:

1. Preheat the oven to 400°F. Peel the outer leaves of the Brussels sprouts and discard them. Add the sprouts to a bowl.

2. Drizzle with oil and toss well to coat in oil. Season with salt. Spread on a baking sheet evenly in one layer. Bake for about 12-15 mins. Take them out from the oven and let them cool.

3. Sprinkle with more salt if you want. Serve topped with smoked paprika.

Nutritional value per serving: Calories 104; Total fat 7 g; Saturated fat 1.4 g; Protein 3 g; Total carbs 9 g; Carbs 5 g; Fiber 4 g; Sugar 1 g

Cheesy crackers

Prep & Cooking Time: 45 mins   Servings: 8

Ingredients:

- ½ cup flax meal
- 1   cup almond flour
- 2   tbsp whole psyllium husks
- 1 cup of water
- 1 cup Parmesan cheese, grated
- 1 tsp salt
- ¼ tsp black pepper

Directions:

1. Mix flax meal, almond flour, psyllium, salt, and pepper in a bowl. Add the cheese to it and mix well. Add water and mix well. Let rest for 15 mins. Preheat the oven to 320°F and divide the dough into 2 parts.

2. Place half of the dough on parchment paper. Place another piece of parchment paper on top and roll the dough out until thin. Cut the dough into 16 equal pieces. Repeat the process with the remaining dough. Bake for 45 mins. Serve.

Nutritional value per serving: Calories 169; Total fat 13.4 g; Saturated fat 2.7 g; Protein 8.4 g; Total carbs 6.3 g; Carbs 1.7 g; Fiber 4.5 g; Sugar 0.8 g

Almond bark

Prep & Cooking time: 15 mins Servings: 20

Ingredients:

- 4 oz. cocoa butter
- ½ cup Swerve sweetener
- ½ tsp vanilla extract
- 2 tbsps water
- ¾ cup cocoa powder
- 1 tbsp butter
- ½ cup powdered Swerve sweetener
- 1½ cups roasted almonds, unsalted
- 2½ oz. unsweetened chocolate, chopped
- ¼ tsp sea salt

Directions:

1. Add 2 tbsps water and ½ cup. Swerve sweetener into a saucepan. Bringthe mixture to a light boil, stirring occasionally. Cook for about 8 to 9 mins until the mixture darkens.

2. Turn the heat off and whisk in 1 tbsp butter. Add 1½ cups roastedalmonds and toss well until coated. Then stir in 2 pinches of salt.

3. Spread almonds onto a parchment-lined baking sheet. Add 4 oz. Cocoabutter and 2½ oz. Unsweetened chocolate to a large saucepan. Melt over medium heat and stir until smooth.

4. Stir in ¾ cup cocoa powder and ½ cup powdered. Swerve sweetener untilsmooth. Turn the heat off and stir in ½ tsp vanilla extract.

5. Reserve 4 tbsps of almonds and keep them aside. Add leftover almondsto the chocolate mixture and stir well.

6. Spread chocolate-almond mixture out onto the same baking sheet. Topwith reserved ¼ cups of almonds and sprinkle with salt.

7. Chill for about 3 hours and then break into chunks. Serve right away!

Nutritional value per serving: Calories 144; Total fat 14 g; Saturated fat 1.3 g; Protein 13 g; Total carbs 5 g; Carbs 2 g; Fiber 3 g; Sugar 10 g

Cheddar jalapeno meatballs

Prep & Cooking Time: 45 mins   Servings: 8

Ingredients:

- 1 ½ lb. Ground beef
- 1 large jalapeno, sliced
- 6 oz sharp cheddar, grated
- ½ cup pork rind crumbs
- 1 egg
- 1   tsp chilli powder
- 2   tbsp cilantro, chopped
- 1 tsp garlic powder
- ½ tsp cumin
- 1 tsp salt and pepper

Directions:

1. Preheat the oven to 375°F and line a rimmed baking sheet withparchment paper.

2. Mix all ingredients in a blender. Blend on high until well combined. Rollthe dough into 1½-inch balls and add to the baking sheet 1 inch apart.

3. Bake for 20 mins. Serve.

Nutritional value per serving: Calories 368; Total fat 24 g; Saturated fat 9.7 g; Protein 33.4 g; Total carbs 1.1 g; Carbs 0.8 g; Fiber 0.3 g; Sugar 1 g

Bacon and fat guacamole bombs Prep &

Cooking Time: 45 mins   Servings: 6

Ingredients:

- ¼ cup butter (softened)
- ½ avocado
- 2 garlic cloves, crushed
- ½ small white onion, diced
- 1 small chilli pepper, finely chopped
- 1   tbsp lime juice
- 2   tbsp cilantro, chopped
- 4 slices bacon
- ¼ tsp sea salt
- Black pepper

Directions:

1.   Preheat the oven to 375°F and line a baking tray with baking paper. Placethe bacon strips on the baking tray.

2.   Bake for 15 mins. Remove the tray from the oven and let cool. Crumblethe bacon.

3.   Cut avocado in half, remove the pit and peel it. Add butter, avocado,chilli pepper, cilantro, crushed garlic, and lime juice to a bowl. Season with salt and pepper. Mash with a fork until combined.

4.   Add onion and mix. Add bacon grease from the baking tray and mixwell. Cover with foil and refrigerate for 30 mins.

5.   Shape the guacamole mixture into 6 balls. Roll each ball into the baconpieces and place on a tray. Serve.

Nutritional value per serving: Calories 156; Total fat 15.2 g; Saturated fat 6.8 g; Protein 3.4 g; Total carbs 2.7 g; Carbs 1.4 g; Fiber 1.3 g; Sugar 0.5 g

Buffalo chicken sausage balls

Prep & Cooking Time: 40 mins   Servings: 12 balls

Ingredients:

- 3 tbsp coconut flour
- 24 oz. bulk chicken sausage
- 1 cup cheddar cheese, shredded
- 1 cup almond flour
- ½ cup Buffalo wing sauce
- ½ tsp cayenne
- 1   tsp salt
- ½ tsp pepper
- 2   garlic cloves, minced
- 1 tsp dried dill
- ⅓ cup mayonnaise
- ⅓ cup almond milk, unsweetened
- ½ tsp dried parsley
- ¼ cup bleu cheese, crumbled
- ½ tsp salt
-   ½ tsp pepper

Directions:

1.   Preheat the oven to 350°F and line 2 baking sheets with parchmentpaper. Mix cheddar cheese, sausage, almond flour, coconut flour, buffalo sauce, cayenne, salt, and pepper in a bowl and mix well until combined. Roll the mixture into 1-inch balls and place on the baking sheets 1 inch apart—Bake for 25 mins.

2.   Mix mayo, almond milk, garlic, parsley, dill, salt, and pepper in a bowl.Mix well and add bleu cheese in. Mix well. Serve balls with the sauce.

Nutritional value per serving: Calories 255; Total fat 19.3 g; Saturated fat 4.7 g; Protein 15.3 g; Total carbs 4.2 g; Carbs 2.5 g; Fiber 1.7 g; Sugar 5 g

Coconut chocolate chip cookies

Prep & Cooking Time: 30 mins   Servings: 6

Ingredients:

- 1 egg
- 3/4 cup coconut shredded
- 1 ¼ cup almond flour
- 1 tsp baking powder
- 1/2 cup swerve sweetener
- 1/2 cup vanilla extract
- 1/2 cup chocolate chips, sugar-free
- 1/2 cup butter
- ¼ tsp fine salt

Directions:

1.   Preheat the oven to 325°F and line a baking sheet with parchment paper.Mix coconut, almond flour, baking powder, and salt in a bowl. Mix butter with sweetener in a separate bowl. Beat in egg and vanilla. Stir to combine. Add this mixture to the flour mixture and beat it well. Add in the chocolate chips.

2.   Shape the dough into 1½-inch balls. Place on the baking sheet 2 inchesapart. Press each ball to ¼-inch thick. Bake for 15 mins. Remove from the oven and cool completely. Serve.

Nutritional value per serving: Calories 268; Total fat 17.4 g; Saturated fat 10.3 g; Protein 12 g; Total carbs 13 g; Carbs 12 g; Fiber 1 g; Sugar 10 g

Creamy Raspberry Cheesecake Bites

Prep& Cooking time: 40 minutes   Servings: 4

Ingredients:

- ¾ cup butter
- 6 drops liquid stevia
- 2 tsp pure vanilla
- ⅛ tsp plus a pinch of sea salt, divided
- 2 tbsps. honey
- ¾ cup raw unsalted cashews
- ¼ cup fresh raspberries, halved (frozen berries work, just thaw and drain them well) ¼ cup raw unsalted pecans
- ⅛ tsp ground cinnamon
-

Directions:

1. Place the butter, stevia, vanilla, and ⅛ tsp salt and blend. Pulse until the mixture is smooth. Scrape down the sides. Add the cashews and process until nuts are broken down to the size of aquarium gravel or smaller.
2. Add the raspberries to a bowl. Stir them by hand, and don't worry if some of them break while others stay whole. Cover and refrigerate for 30 minutes. The mixture will become firm. Grind the pecans into a near flour-like state. Add cinnamon and salt.
3. Remove the batter from the refrigerator. Scoop out a tbsp of the cheesecake mixture with a melon baller. While the batter is still in the melon baller, press the open end into the pecan dust. This is the flat side. Release the batter with the flat side down on a plate. You have just made a cheesecake bite. Before serving, put in the refrigerator for about an hour.

Nutrition value per serving: calories 33, fat 1g, fibre 1g, carbs 6g, Protein 2g

Decadent Cherry Chocolate Almond Clusters

Prep & Cooking time: 35 minutes   Servings: 5

Ingredients:

- 1 tbsp. smooth nut butter of your choice
- 8 ounces dark chocolate
- 1 cup oats
- ⅓ cup raw unsalted nuts, chopped
- ⅓ cup dried, unsweetened cherries or raisins, chopped

<u>Directions</u>:

1 Boil water and simmer and then add the nut butter and chocolate, occasionally stirring for two to three minutes. Take out from heat and stir in the oats, nuts, and dried fruit.
2. Stripe a baking sheet with wax or parchment paper. Drib the batter by rounded teaspoonful onto the baking sheet, making 20 mounds.
3. Abode the baking sheet in the refrigerator for 25 minutes or until the mounds set. Remove and store in an airtight container.

Nutrition value per serving: calories 260, fat 25g, fibre 2g, carbs 8g, Protein 2g

Low-carb waffles

Prep & Cooking time: 30 minutes   Servings: 4

Ingredients

- 6 eggs
- 2 mashed bananas
- Unsweetened almond butter two tsp.
- Quinoa flour three tsp.
- Salt quarter tsp.
- Cinnamon powder half tsp.
- Olive oil extra virgin half tsp.
- Coconut butter half tbsp.
- Almond butter half tbsp.
- Sliced quarter banana
- Walnuts chopped half tbsp.
- Maple syrup one tbsp.

Directions

1. Plugin the waffle maker and let it heat up. Get a mixing container and in it, mix the bananas mashed, eggs, quinoa flour, cinnamon, unsweetened almond butter, and salt until you get a smooth mixture.
2. When the waffle maker is hot enough, use the extra virgin olive oil to grease it. Divide the waffle mixture into three portions and cook each

until it is ready. Remove and do the same for the remaining mixture as well.

3. When cooled off, top the waffles with the remaining almond butter, quarter sliced bananas, and walnuts, chopped maple syrup, and coconut butter.

Nutrition value per serving: calories 200, fat 8g, fibre 2g, carbs 8g, Protein 6g

Bacon tacos

Prep & Cooking time: 30 minutes   Servings: 4

Ingredients

- 14 pieces halved bacon
- An avocado seeded, peeled and sliced
- Black pepper powder quarter tsp.
- Monterey jack shredded in half a cup
- 5 eggs
- Fresh chives chopped two tbsp.
- Almond milk one tbsp.
- A pinch of salt
- Unsweetened butter one tbsp.
- A little hot sauce

Directions

1. Begin by preparing the taco shells first. Heat the oven in advance at 400c.
2. Get a baking sheet and line the inside with foil. Place the bacon strips in it, crisscrossing each other to form a square at the end. Do this again to form three consecutive weaves.
3. Take the black pepper powder and season the arranged bacon pieces, and press flat the bacon using a baking rack that is inverted. Place the sheet for baking in the oven that you heated in advance and let the bacon bake until it is crispy, which will take half an hour.

4. When the bacon is ready, using a knife for paring, cut up the crispy bacon squares to form small circles, which will be the taco shells. This should be done very fast.

5 Get the eggs and crack them in a mixing container. Add the almond milk and whisk both until they are well mixed. Take a frying pan and, over medium heat, melt the unsweetened butter.

6. Follow this by pouring the whisked egg mixture and slowly move the eggs around to turn them into scrambled eggs. Add salt and black pepper powder for seasoning followed by chives, then remove the frying pan from the heat.

7. Get a plate that you will use to serve and arrange the bacon taco shells on top of it. Add the scrambled eggs on top of the bacon taco shells, then add a little cheese, avocado slices, and a little hot sauce as well.

Nutrition value per serving: calories 260, fat 8g, fibre 2g, carbs 8g, Protein 45g

Eggs with cauliflower

Prep & Cooking time: 30 minutes   Servings: 4

Ingredients

- 1/2 a Cauliflower head
- Olive oil extra virgin one tbsp.
- 3 eggs
- Black pepper freshly ground quarter tsp.
- Salt quarter tsp.
- Cornstarch quarter tsp.
- Cheddar cheese shredded one cup
- Bacon two slices Paprika two tsp.
- Fresh chives one tsp.
-

Directions

1. Get a box grater, and with it, grate the half head of cauliflower until it is well grated. Place the grated cauliflower into a mixing container

and add an egg to it together with the cheddar cheese that has been shredded, cornstarch, and salt. Mix them all well.

2. Get a large frying pan and heat the olive oil over medium heat. Using a serving spoon, scoop the cauliflower mix into the frying pan and

shape it into patties. Cook these patties for five minutes until they are crispy and done. Ensure to flip both sides.

3. Get a saucepan and poach the remaining two eggs over medium heat using boiling water. Get another pan for frying and over a medium flame, let the olive oil become hot. Follow this by adding in bacon pieces and allow them to cook until they are crispy. Crack the eggs and remove them from the shell. Slice them into circles.

4. Place the cooked cauliflower patties on a plate and add the sliced eggs together with the slices of crispy bacon. Sprinkle the paprika and chives and serve.

Nutrition value per serving: calories 40, fat 1g, fibre 2g, carbs 8g, Protein 2g

Bacon with Brussels sprouts and eggs

Prep & Cooking time: 30 minutes   Servings: 4

Ingredients

- 6 eggs large
- Trimmed and halved Brussels sprouts one cup
- Quarter tsp. black pepper freshly ground
- Bacon 6 slices
- Salt quarter tsp.
- Olive oil extra virgin two tbsp.
- Buffalo sauce three tbsp.
- Flakes of red pepper quarter tsp.
- Powder of garlic half tsp.
- Fresh chives chopped one tsp.

Directions

1. Heat your oven in advance at 425c. Get a mixing container and in it, mix the halved Brussels sprouts, powder of garlic, flakes of red pepper, bacon, buffalo sauce, and olive oil.

2   Add the black pepper that has been freshly ground and the salt to season the mix. Get a large baking sheet and cover it with the mixture evenly.

3   Place the large baking sheet into the oven you heated in advance and let it bake for fifteen minutes when the bacon will be crispy and the Brussels sprouts tender. Take the sheet out and use a wooden spoon to make six holes in the baked mixture.

4. Crack the eggs and pour in the holes you made using the wooden spoon and sprinkle a little black pepper that has been freshly ground and salt to season the eggs. Return the baking sheet into the oven and bake for ten minutes until the eggs are done. Take the baking sheet out of the oven and sprinkle the fresh chives and buffalo sauce on top before serving.

Nutrition value per serving: calories 100, fat 7g, fibre 2g, carbs 8g, Protein 6g

IF poultry and meat recipes (at least 10)

Warming Lamb Stew

Prep & Cooking time:1 hour 35 minutes   Servings: 7

Ingredients

- 2 tsp olive oil, extra virgin is best
- 1lb lamb, make sure it is as lean as you can get it, and cut into cubes
- A little salt
- A little pepper
- 1 large onion, chopped
- 1   celery stalk, chopped
- 2   garlic cloves, chopped
- 2 carrots, cut into small pieces
- 1.5tsp oregano
- 2 cups broth, chicken broth, works best here, but you can use vegetable also
- 0.25 cup red wine, the dry version works well
- 1 x 15oz can of tomato sauce, the smoother, the better
- 1 tsp zest from a lemon
- 0.5 tsp cinnamon
- 1 sweet potato, chopped
- 1 lemon, chopped

Direction

1. You will need a Dutch oven for this recipe, and you need to add the oil and set it to medium to high heat. Once heated up, add the meat and add a little salt and pepper to your taste.
2. Sear the lamb on both sides. Now, add the celery and the onion and cook for around 4 minutes, until soft. Add the garlic and cook for half a minute. Add the oregano and combine well, and then add the carrots, stirring all the while for another half a minute.
3 Add the wine, the broth, the tomato sauce, the lemon zest, and the cinnamon and combine everything well. Next, add the sweet potato and the lemon and combine once more.

4 Allow the mixture to reach the boiling point and then turn the heat down to a lower temperature, covering over and allowing to simmer. Cook until the vegetables are soft and the lamb is totally cooked for between 80-90 minutes. You may need to add more salt and pepper, according to your personal preferences.

Nutrition value per serving: calories 280, fat 8g, fibre 2g, carbs 7g, Protein 8g

Spicy Chicken Masala

Prep & Cooking time: 30 minutes   Servings: 4

Ingredients

- 4 chicken cutlets, pounded until they are quite thin
- A little salt to taste
- 1   egg, beaten
- 0.5 cup of whole-wheat flour, plus another 1.5 tbsp
- 2   x 8oz packs of button mushrooms, sliced
- 4 cloves of garlic, minced
- 0.5 cup Marsala wine, the dry version works best
- 1 cup of chicken broth, low fat is best
- 0.25 cup of Greek yoghurt
- A little black pepper
- Cheese for topping if you want to

Direction

1. You will need two non-stick pans for this recipe, and they both need to be placed over medium to low heat. Season your chicken with a little salt and wait for the pans to heat up, spraying with a little cooking oil
2. In a small mixing bowl, add the beaten egg and the half cup of wholewheat flour and mix together. Dip the chicken into the mixture and cover completely before placing it into the pans, two in each. Cook the chicken for about 4 minutes on each side and then
3. Place the chicken onto a plate and keep warm with aluminium foil.

Clean the pans out and turn the heat up, adding a little more spray to the pans

4. Place one package of mushrooms into each pan and cook for around 3 minutes. Now place all the mushrooms in one pan and add the garlic and a little salt. Turn the heat down and cook for one more minute. Add the rest of the whole-wheat flour to the mixture, along with the wine and the broth, combining everything well. Allow the mixture to simmer for around 3 minutes.

5. Take the pan off the heat and add the yoghurt and a little more salt and pepper, stirring well. Remove the foil from the chicken and place it on a serving plate, pouring the Marsala sauce over the top. Add a little cheese to melt on top if you like

Nutrition value per serving: calories 340, fat 15g, fibre 2g, carbs 18g, Protein 30g

Quick Ratatouille

Prep & Cooking time: 25 minutes   Servings: 4

Ingredients

- 2 onions, sliced
- 4 cloves of garlic, chopped very finely
- 0.5 cup olive oil
- 1 green pepper, cut into small pieces
- 1 red pepper, cut into small pieces
- 1 aubergine (eggplant), cut into cubes
- 4 zucchinis, cubed
- 8 tomatoes, seeded and chopped
- 1   tbsp basil, shredded. Fresh is best but if you have to go with dried,just use 1 tsp)
- 1.5 tsp salt
- A little black pepper

Direction

1 You will need a large and deep-frying pan or saucepan, Add the oil and allow to reach a medium to high heat. Add the onions and the garlic, and cook for a few minutes until the onions are clear.

2 Add the peppers, zucchini, and the aborigine (eggplant) and combine. Turn the heat down and play over the pan, allowing it to simmer for around 10 minutes. Add the salt and pepper, as well as the tomatoes and stir well, covering the pan once more and allowing it to continue cooking for another 10 minutes.

3. Take the lid off the pan and stir the mixture, allowing it to reduce. Add a little salt and pepper and serve whilst still warm. The mixture is done when it is blended well but isn't particularly 'wet.'

Nutrition value per serving: calories 270, fat 8g, fibre 2g, carbs 8g, Protein 6g

Cajun Chicken with Buckwheat Crust

Prep & Cooking time: 30 minutes   Servings: 4

Ingredients

- 0.25 cup buckwheat flour
- 2 tbsp paprika powder, the sweet version is the best for this recipe
- 1 tsp turmeric powder
- 1 tsp cumin powder
- 1 tsp coriander powder
- A little salt
- A little pepper
- 0.5 tsp cinnamon powder
- A little coconut oil for cooking
- 4 chicken breasts, but you can use thighs if you prefer
- 1 red chilli pepper, chopped very finely (be careful to wash your hands!)
- A few almonds, chopped very finely

Direction

1. Take a mixing bowl and combine the flour and the powders. Take your chicken and coat evenly with the mixture. Take a large frying pan and add the coconut oil, allowing it to heat up over a medium to low heat

2. Place the chicken in the pan and cook on both sides until completely cooked through. Once cooked, transfer to a serving plate and serve with the finely chopped chilli and the almonds
3. Add a little salt and pepper according to your personal preference

Nutrition value per serving: calories 345, fat 8g, fibre 2g, carbs 8g, Protein 45g

Butter Chicken

Prep & Cooking time: 35 minutes   Servings: 4

Ingredients:

- Butter – ¼ cup
- Mushrooms – 2 cups, sliced
- Chicken thighs – 4 large
- Onion powder – ½ tsp
- Garlic powder – ½ tsp
- Kosher salt – 1 tsp
- Black pepper – ¼ tsp
- Water – ½ cup
- Dijon mustard – 1 tsp
- Fresh tarragon – 1 tbsp., chopped

Directions:

1. Season the chicken thighs with onion powder, garlic powder, salt, and pepper. In a sauté pan, melt 1 tbsp. Butter.
2. Sear the chicken thighs for about 3 to 4 minutes per side, or until both sides are golden brown. Rem hve the thighs from the pan. Add the remaining 3 tbsp of butter to the pan and melt. Add the mushrooms and cook for 4 to 5 minutes or until golden brown.
3. Add the Dijon mustard and water to the pan. Stir to deglaze. Place the chicken thighs back in the pan with the skin side up. Cover and simmer for 15 minutes.
4. Stir in the fresh herbs. Let sit for 5 minutes and serve.

Nutrition value per serving: Calories 414 Total Fat 32.9g Saturated Fat

13.6g Cholesterol 149mg Sodium 786mg Total Carbohydrate 2g Dietary Fiber 0.5g Total Sugars 0.8g Protein 26.5g

Lamb Curry

Prep& Cooking time:4 hours 10 minutes   Servings: 6

Ingredients:

- Fresh ginger – 2 tbsp. grated
- Garlic – 2 cloves, peeled and minced
- Cardamom – 2 tsp
- Onion – 1 peeled and hopped
- Cloves – 6
- Lamb meat – 1 pound, cubed
- Cumin powder – 2 tsp
- Garam masala – 1 tsp
- Chili powder – ½ tsp
- Turmeric – 1 tsp
- Coriander – 2 tsp
- Spinach – 1 pound
- Canned – 14 ounces

Directions:

1. In a slow cooker, mix lamb with tomatoes, spinach, ginger, garlic, onion, cardamom, cloves, cumin, garam masala, chilli, turmeric, and coriander.
2. Stir well—cover and cook on high for 4 hours. Uncover the slow cooker, stir the chilli, divide into bowls, and serve.

Nutrition value per serving: Calories 186 Total Fat 7.2g Saturated Fat 2.5g Cholesterol 38mg Sodium 477mg Total Carbohydrate 16.3g Dietary Fiber 5g Total Sugars 5g Protein 14.4g.

Garlic Herb Grilled Chicken Breast Prep &

Cooking time: 30 minutes   Servings: 4

Ingredients:

- Chicken Breasts, skinless and boneless - 1¼ pounds.
- Olive oil - 2 teaspoons.
- Garlic & Herb Seasoning Blend - 1
- tablespoon. Salt and Pepper **Directions**:

1. Pat dry the chicken breasts, coat them with olive oil and season them with salt and pepper on both sides. Season the chicken with garlic and herb seasoning or any other seasoning of your choice. Turn the grill on and oil the grate.
2. Place the chicken on the hot grate and let it grill till the sides turn white. Flip them over and let it cook again. When the internal temperature is about 160 degree, it is most likely cooked. Set aside for 15 minutes. Chop into pieces.

Nutritional value per serving: Calories: 187, Fats: 6g, Protein: 32g, Carbs: 5g

Paprika Lamb Chops

Prep & Cooking time: 25 minutes   Servings: 4

Ingredients:

- 2   lamb racks, cut into chops
- 3   tablespoons paprika
- ¾ cup cumin powder
- 1 teaspoon chili powder, Salt and pepper to taste

Directions:

1. Take a bowl and add paprika, cumin, chilli, salt, pepper, and stir. Add lamb chops and rub the mixture. Heat grill over medium-temperature and add lamb chops, cook for 5 minutes. Flip and cook for 5 minutes more, flip again. Cook for 2 minutes, flip and cook for 2 minutes more. Serve and enjoy!

Nutrition value per serving: Calories: 200 Fat: 5g Carbohydrates: 4g Protein: 8g

Delicious Tur

Prep & Cooking time: 20 minutes   Servings: 6

Ingredients:

- 1 and a ¼ pounds of ground turkey, lean - 4 green onions, minced
- 1   tablespoon of olive oil - 1 garlic clove, minced
- 2   teaspoon of chilli paste
- 8-ounce water chestnut, diced
- 3   tablespoon of hoisin sauce
- 2 tablespoon of coconut aminos
- 1 tablespoon of rice vinegar
- 12 butter lettuce leaves
- 1/8 teaspoon of salt

Directions:

1. Take a pan and place it over medium heat; add turkey and garlic to the pan. Heat for 6 minutes until cooked. Take a bowl and transfer turkey to the bowl. Add onions and water chestnuts
2. Stir in hoisin sauce, coconut aminos, vinegar, and chilli paste. Toss well and transfer the mix to lettuce leaves. Serve and enjoy!

Nutrition value per serving: Calories: 162 Fat: 4g Net Carbohydrates: 7g Protein: 23g

Bacon and Chicken Garlic Wrap

Prep & Cooking time: 25 minutes   Servings: 4

Ingredients:

- 1 chicken fillet, cut into small cubes
- 8-9 thin slices bacon, cut to fit cubes
- 6 garlic cloves, minced

Directions:

1. Preheat your oven to 400 degrees F. Line a baking tray with aluminium foil. Add minced garlic to a bowl and rub each chicken piece with it. Wrap bacon piece around each garlic chicken bite
2. Transfer bites to the baking sheet, keeping a little bit of space between them. Bake for about 15-20 minutes until crispy. Serve and enjoy!

Nutrition value per serving: Calories: 260 Fat: 19g Carbohydrates: 5g Protein: 22g

IF salad and soups recipes (at least 10)

Caesar salad

Prep& Cooking Time: 15 mins   Servings: 4

Ingredients:

- 2 chicken breasts, grilles and 1 head romaine lettuce, chopped
- 2   cup grape tomatoes, halved and parmesan cheese stripsFor

the Dressing:

- 3   garlic clove, minced and 1/2 lemon, juiced
- 1 1/2 tsp Dijon mustard
- 3/4 cup mayonnaise and 1 1/2 tsp anchovy paste
- 1 tsp Worchestershire sauce and salt and pepper, to taste

Directions:

1. Mix all the dressing ingredients in a bowl and whisk well to combine. Cover and refrigerate the salad dressing. Mix grape tomatoes, romaine lettuce and cooked chicken in a bowl. Crumble the cheese crisps into smaller pieces. Add dressing on top. Toss to combine and serve.

Nutritional value per serving: Calories 400; Total fat 25 g; Saturated fat 12 g; Protein 33 g; Total carbs 9 g; Carbs 5 g; Fiber 4 g; Sugar 4 g

Thai beef salad

Prep & Cooking Time: 15 mins   Servings: 4

Ingredients:

- 1½ lb. flank steak
- 1 tbsp olive oil and 1 tsp sea salt
- 1 cup cucumbers, chopped
- 1 head lettuce, chopped and 1 cup grape tomatoes, halved
- ¼ cup basil, cut into ribbons and ¼ cup cilantro, chopped
- ¼ cup red onion, sliced
- ¼ cup olive oil and ¼ cup coconut aminos

- 1   tbsp fish sauce
- 2   tbsp lime juice and 1 tbsp Thai red curry paste**Directions**:

1.   Mix oil, coconut aminos, fish sauce, lime juice, and curry paste in a bowland whisk to combine. Season steak with salt on all sides. Put steak slices in a single layer into a glass baking dish. Add half of the marinade over the steak.

2.   Cover meat with plastic wrap and refrigerate for 8 hours. Cover thereserved dressing and refrigerate. Mix lettuce, cucumbers, grape tomatoes, cilantro, red onion, and basil in a bowl. Cook beef in a hot pan until brown on all sides. Let beef rest for 5 mins. Slice against the grain. Serve salad with beef and dressing.

Nutritional value per serving: Calories 426; Total fat 26 g; Saturated fat 14.2 g; Protein 38 g; Total carbs 8 g; Carbs 7 g; Fiber 1 g; Sugar 2 g

Zucchini noodle salad

Prep & Cooking Time: 15 mins   Servings: 8 cups

Ingredients:

- 8 oz. mozzarella pearls
- 1 oz. basil, chopped
- 4 zucchinis, spiralized
- 4 oz. cherry tomatoes, sliced in half
- 3 tbsp red wine vinegar
- ¼ cup extra virgin olive oil
- 1 tbsp lemon juice and ¼ tsp garlic powder
- ½ tsp salt and ¼ tsp pepper

Directions:

1. Whisk red wine, oil, lemon juice, garlic powder, salt, and pepper in a bowl. Add the remaining ingredients to a bowl and add dressing on top. Toss well to combine. Serve.

Nutritional value per serving: Calories 186; Total fat 13 g; Saturated fat 4 g; Protein 7 g; Total carbs 4 g; Carbs 3 g; Fiber 1 g; Sugar 3 g

Kale and Brussels sprout salad

Prep & Cooking Time: 15 mins

Servings: 8

Ingredients:

- ½ lb. Brussels sprouts, outer leaves and stems removed
- ½ bunch curly kale
- 6 slices cooked bacon
- ½ cup dried cranberries
- ½ cup walnuts
- 2 tbsps lemon juice
- ⅓ cup olive oil
- ½ tsp garlic powder
- 1 tbsp Dijon mustard
- ¼ tsp sea salt
- ¼ tsp black pepper

Directions:

1. Add Brussels sprouts to a blender and blend well until chopped. Add kale leaves to it and pulse until shredded.
2. Whisk mustard, olive oil, lemon juice, garlic powder, salt, and pepper in a bowl until well mixed.
3. Add kale and Brussels sprouts and stir to combine. Add the cooked bacon, walnuts, and cranberries in it. Toss well. Serve.

Nutritional value per serving: Calories 192; Total fat 17 g; Saturated fat 1.6 g; Protein 6 g; Total carbs 6 g; Carbs 4 g; Fiber 2 g; Sugar 3 g

Cabbage coconut salad

Prep & Cooking Time: 5 mins   Servings: 4

Ingredients:

- ¼ cup of coconut oil

- ½ head white cabbage, shredded
- 1 lemon juice and ⅓ cup dried coconut, unsweetened
- ¼ cup tamari sauce and ½ tsp ginger, dried
- 3 tsp sesame seeds
- ½ tsp curry powder
- ½ tsp cumin

Directions:

1. Add all the ingredients to a bowl and toss well. Cover and refrigerate for 1 hour. Serve.

Nutritional value per serving: Calories 309; Total fat 5 g; Saturated fat 8 g; Protein 12 g; Total carbs 12 g; Carbs 6 g; Fiber 6 g; Sugar 3 g

Grilled chicken salad

Prep& Cooking Time: 20 mins   Servings: 2

Ingredients:

- ½ lb chicken thigh, grilled and sliced and 1 tsp fresh thyme
- 4 cups romaine lettuce, chopped
- 2   garlic cloves, crushed and ¼ cup cherry tomatoes, chopped
- 3   tbsp extra virgin olive oil and ½ cucumber thinly sliced
- 2 tbsp red wine vinegar and ½ avocado, sliced 1
- oz olives, pitted and sliced and 1 oz Feta cheese
- salt and pepper **Directions**:

1. Season chicken with a tsp of thyme, crushed garlic, pepper, and salt. Preheat oil in a pan over medium heat. Cook chicken until golden brown. Mix olives, sliced cucumber, chopped lettuce, sliced avocado, and ¼ cup tomatoes in a large bowl.

2. Add chicken to the salad. Sprinkle with crumbled cheese. Drizzle witholive oil and vinegar. Enjoy!

Nutritional value per serving: Calories 617; Total fat 52 g; Saturated fat 4 g; Protein 30 g; Total carbs 11 g; Carbs 7 g; Fiber 4 g; Sugar 2.5 g

Pasta Bolognese Soup

Prep & Cooking time: 45 minutes   Servings: 5

Ingredients

- 2 tsp olive oil and 3 onions, chopped finely
- 2 carrots, peeled and chopped finely
- 2 celery stick, chopped finely and 3 cloves of garlic, chopped finely
- 250g of lean steak/beef mince and 500g pasta
- 1 tbsp vegetable stock and 1 tsp paprika, smoked works well
- 4 pieces of thyme, fresh and 100mg penne, wholemeal and 45g

parmesan cheese, grated finely **Direction**

1. Take a large pan and add the oil, heat over a medium heat. Add the onions and cook until translucent. Add the carrots, garlic, and celery, cooking for 5 minutes, Add the mince to the pan and break it up well. Once the mince has browned, add the stock and the passata, adding 1 litre of hot water
2. Stir well, and then add the thyme and paprika, combining once more. Add the lid to the pan and allow to simmer for 15 minutes, Add the penne and stir through, cooking for another 165 minutes. Add the cheese and stir. Serve in bowls whilst still warm

Nutrition value per serving: calories 182, fat 4g, fibre 2g, carbs 14g, Protein 3g

Potato and Beef Soup

Prep & Cooking time: 1 hour 10 minutes   Servings: 6

Ingredients:

- Cooking spray and Cumin (0.5 tsp.)
- Chopped cilantro (2 tbsps.)
- Red or Yukon Gold potatoes (1.5 cups)
- Water (1.5 cup) Diced tomatoes (2 cups)
- Diced onion (1 pcs.) Beef sirloin steak (0.5 lb.)

Directions

1. Rinse off the beefsteak and blot it dry. Slice into smaller cubes and set aside.

2. Coat the inside of a heavy stew pot with some cooking spray and place it on the hot stove for about a minute to heat-up the pot.
3. Add the prepared beef to the stew pot and cook until the pieces are browned all over. This will take about five minutes. Stir in the onion and let it cook until tender.
4. Stir in the water, cumin, and tomatoes. Mix this well and bring it to a boil. Once at a boil, reduce the heat to medium, and cover and let simmer for about 20 minutes.
5. Uncover the pot and then stir in the cubed potatoes. Cover this and let it simmer for a bit longer until both the beef and the potatoes are tender, which will take another 10 minutes.
6. At this time, turn the heat off and let it stand, with the cover on, for about 5 minutes. Ladle this into some soup bowls and then serve.

Nutrition value per serving: calories 555, fat 28g, fibre 2g, carbs 6g, Protein 67g

Dieter's chicken soup

Prep& Cooking Time:1 hour 10 minutes   Servings: 8

Ingredients:

- 2 quarts sodium-free or light Chicken broth
- 1   pkg shredded Cabbage
- 2   cups Celery, diced
- 1 large Onion, diced
- 1   large Tomato, diced
- 2   boneless, skinless chicken breasts, diced
- 1 Tablespoon ground Thyme
- 1 teaspoon ground sweet Basil Black pepper

Direction

1. Add all ingredients to a large stockpot. Cook until tender.

Nutrition value per serving: calories 200, fat 8g, fibre 2g, carbs 8g, Protein 6g

Gingered carrot soup

Prep & Cooking Time: 45 minutes   Servings: 5

Ingredients:

- 3 Tablespoons unsalted Butter
- 1 cup Leeks, sliced (or white onion)
- 1 Tablespoon fresh ginger, peeled and minced
- 1   ½ lb (~9) Carrots, peeled, cut into 1" lengths
- 2   cups Chicken stock or low-sodium Chicken broth
- 2 cups freshly squeezed Orange juice
- ¼ cup chopped fresh Mint Salt, to taste Ground White Pepper, to taste

Direction

1. In a soup pot, melt butter over medium-high heat. Add the leek and ginger, and sauté until the leek is tender but not browned (about five minutes). Add the carrots, and sauté until coated with butter. Stir in the stock or broth, and bring to a boil. Reduce the heat to low, cover, and simmer until the carrots are very tender (about 30 minutes).
2. Working in batches, if necessary, transfers the soup to a food processor or blender and puree until smooth. Add the orange juice, and blend well. Stir in the chopped mint, and season to taste with salt and pepper.

Nutrition value per serving: calories 624, fat 8g, fibre 2g, carbs 8g, Protein 17g

Great vegetable soup

Prep & Cooking Time: 55 minutes   Servings: 6

Ingredients:

- 1, 15-ounce can Whole Tomatoes, chopped
- 1 medium Onion, chopped and 3 large Garlic cloves, minced 3-
- 4 Celery stalks, chopped

- 1 Tablespoon dried Parsley and 1 teaspoon dried Marjoram 5
- cups Broccoli and other vegetables, such as carrots, cauliflower, zucchini, peppers, leeks, potatoes, turnips, and corn. And 6 cups Water
- 6 teaspoon low salt Bouillon or 5 Bouillon cubes, any flavor and ½ teaspoon Black pepper
- 1 cup uncooked Macaroni or Shells Grated cheese, optional **Direction**

1. In a soup pot, combine tomatoes, onion, garlic, celery, parsley and marjoram. Place over medium heat and sauté frequently stirring until celery and onion are soft (about 20 min). Watch carefully to ensure juice doesn't boil away. If it gets low, add a little water. Meanwhile, dice vegetable into half-inch cubes. Add water, bouillon, vegetables, and pepper.
2. Cover and bring to a boil. Adjust heat and simmer briskly, partially covered for 10 minutes, stirring once or twice. Stir in macaroni and simmer until pasta is tender. Let rest 10 minutes, serve in soup bowls. Top with cheese

Nutrition value per serving: calories 280, fat 18g, fibre 2g, carbs 18g, Protein 10g

IF fish and seafood recipes (at least 10)

Roasted Fish with Vegetables

Prep & Cooking: 45 minutes   Serving 2-3

Ingredients

• Four skinless salmon fillets: 5-6 ounces

• Two red, yellow, orange sweet peppers, cut into rings

• Five cloves of garlic chopped

• Sea salt: half tsp and Olive oil: 2 tbsp.

• Black pepper: half tsp and Pitted halved olives: ¼ cup

- One lemon and Parsley: 1 and ½ cups

- Finely snipped fresh oregano:1/4 cup**Directions**

    1. Let the oven preheat to 425 F. Put the potatoes in a bowl. Drizzle 1 spoon of oil, sprinkle with salt (1/8 tsp.), and garlic. Mix well, shift to the baking pan, cover with foil. Roast them for half an hour
    2. In the meantime, thaw the salmon. Combine the sweet peppers, parsley, oregano, olives, salt (1/8 tsp) and pepper in the same bowl. Add one tablespoon of oil, mix well.
    3. Wash salmon and dry it with paper towels. Sprinkle with salt (1/4 Tsp), Black pepper, and top of it, salmon. Uncover it and roast for ten minutes or till salmon starts to flake.
    4. Add lemon zest and lemon juice over salmon and vegetables. Serve hot

Nutrition value Per Serving: 278 calories| total fat 12 g | carbohydrates 9.2 g| protein 15.4 g | Cholesterol 7.1 mg| Sodium 131 mg| potassium 141 mg| Phosphorus 121 mg

Salmon with Brussel Sprout

Prep & Cooking: 30 minutes   Serving 2

Ingredients

- Steamed Brussels: 1 cup and Fresh salmon: 4 ounces

- Light soy sauce: 2 tablespoons

- Dijon mustard: 1 and 1/2 tablespoons

- Salt & pepper, to taste

Directions

1. Let the broiler pre-heat. Cover the salmon surface with mustard and soy sauce. Spray the baking sheet with foil, put salmon in the baking pan, and broil for ten minutes, or until salmon is completely cooked through. Meanwhile, steam the Brussel sprout, if not already steamed. Serve salmon and sprinkle salt & pepper to taste.

Nutrition value per serving: Calories 236|Protein 15.3 g |Carbohydrates 7.2 g| Fat 16.4 g| Cholesterol 8.9 mg| Sodium 143 mg| potassium 176 mg| Phosphorus 132 mg

Charred Shrimp & Pesto Buddha Bowls

Prep & Cooking: 45 minutes   Serving 4

Ingredients

• Pesto: 1/3 cup and Vinegar: 2 tbsp.

• Olive oil: 1 tbsp and Salt: 1/8 tsp.

• Ground pepper: ¼ tsp and Peeled & deveined large shrimp: one pound

• Arugula: 4 cups and Cooked quinoa: 2 cups**Directions**

1. In a large bowl, mix pesto, oil, vinegar, salt, and pepper. Take out four tbsp of mixture in another bowl.
2. Place skillet over medium flame. Add shrimp, let it cook for five minutes, stirring, until only charred a little. move to a plate
3. Use the vinaigrette to mix with quinoa and arugula in a bowl. Divide the mixture of the arugula into four bowls. Cover with shrimp, add 1 tbsp. Of the pesto mixture to each bowl, and serve.

Nutrition value Per Serving: 329 calories| total fat 18 g | carbohydrates 17.2 g| protein 17 g | Cholesterol 6.7 mg| Sodium 154 mg| potassium 143 mg| Phosphorus 123 mg

Cilantro-Lime Swordfish

Prep & Cooking: 35 minutes   Serving 2-3

Ingredients

• Swordfish: 1 pound and Half cup of low-fat mayonnaise

• Lime juice: 2 tablespoons and Half cup of fresh cilantro**Directions**

1. In a bowl, mix chopped cilantro, lime juice, low-fat mayonnaise mix well. Take ¼ cup from the mix and leave the rest aside

2. Apply the rest of the mayo mix to the fish with a brush. In a skillet, over medium heat, spray oil
3. Add fish fillets, cook for 8 minutes, turning once, or until fish is cooked to your liking. Serve with sauce.

Nutrition value per serving: Calories 292 | Protein 20 g |Carbohydrates 1 g| Fat 23 g| Cholesterol 57 mg| Sodium 228 mg| Potassium 237 mg| Phosphorus 128 mg

Pesto-Crusted Catfish

Prep & Cooking: 25 minutes   Serving 4

Ingredients

• Pesto: 4 teaspoons and Catfish: 2 pounds (no bones)

• Panko bread crumbs: ¾ cup

• Olive oil: 2 tablespoons and Half cup of vegan cheese

• Seasoning Blend: (No salt added spices)
• Red pepper flakes: half teaspoon and Garlic powder, low sodium: 1teaspoon

• Dried oregano: half teaspoon and Black pepper: half teaspoon

• Onion powder: 1 teaspoon**Directions**

1. Let the oven preheat to 400 F. In a bowl, add all the seasoning, sprinkle over fish on both sides.
2. Then spread pesto on each side of fish. In a bowl, mix bread crumbs, cheese, oil—coat pesto fish in crumbs mix. Spray oil on the baking tray. Add fish on a baking tray. Bake at 400° F for 20 minutes or until it's ready.
3. Let it rest for ten minutes. Then serve.

Nutrition value Per Serving: Calories 312 | total Fat 16 g | Cholesterol 83 mg| Sodium 272 mg| Carbohydrates 15 g| Protein 26 g| Phosphorus 417 mg| Potassium 576 mg|

Sesame-Seared Salmon

Prep& Cooking Time: 25 Minutes   Servings: 4

Ingredients:

- 4 wild salmon fillets (about 1lb.)
- 1½ tbsps. of sesame seeds
- 2 tbsps. of toasted sesame oil
- 1½ tbsps. of avocado oil and 1 tsp. of sea salt

Directions:

1.   Using a paper towel or a clean kitchen towel, pat the fillets to dry. Brusheach with a tablespoon of sesame oil and season with a half teaspoon of salt. Place a large skillet over medium-high heat and drizzle with avocado oil. Once the oil is hot, add the salmon fillets with the flesh side down— Cook for about 3 minutes and flip. Cook the skin side for an additional 3-4 minutes without overcooking it.

2.   Remove the pan from the heat and brush with the remaining sesame oil.Season with the remaining salt and sprinkle with sesame seeds. Best served with a green salad.

Nutrition value per serving: Calories: 198, Fat: 12g, Fiber: 2g, Carbs: 20g, Protein: 5g

Thai Fish Curry

Prep & Cooking time: 15mins   Serves: 6

Ingredients:

- 1   1/3 cup Olive oil and 1 ½ pound Salmon fillets
- 2   cups Coconut milk, freshly squeezed
- 2 tablespoons Curry powder
- 1 ¼ cup Cilantro chopped

Directions:

1. In your instant pot, add in all ingredients. Apply a seasoning of pepper and salt.

2. Give a good stir.
3. Set the lid in place and the vent to point to "Sealing."
4. Set the IP to "Manual" and cook for 10 minutes.
5. Do quick pressure release.

Nutrition value per serving: Calories: 470 Carbs: 5,6 g Protein: 25,5 g Fat: 39,8 g

Bonus Intermittent Fasting Recipes

Beet Blast Smoothie

Prep & Cooking time: 5 minutes   Servings: 1

Ingredients:

- 1½ cup unsweetened plant-based milk
- 1 Granny Smith apple, peeled, cored, and chopped
- 1 cup chopped frozen beets and 1 cup frozen blueberries
- ½ cup frozen cherries and ¼-inch fresh ginger root, peeled

Directions:

1. In a blender, combine all the ingredients and blend until smooth.
2. Serve immediately or store in the freezer in a resalable jar.

Nutrition value per serving: Calories: 324 Total fat: 5 g Carbohydrates: 70 g Fiber: 15 g

Protein: 5 g Calcium: 72% Vitamin D: 38% Vitamin B12: 0% Iron: 15% Zinc: 4%

Green Power Smoothie

Prep & Cooking time:15 minutes   Servings: 1

Ingredients:

- 3 cups fresh spinach and 1½ cup frozen pineapple
- 1 cup unsweetened plant-based milk
-

1 cup fresh kale and 1 Granny Smith apple, peeled, cored, and chopped
- ½ small avocado, pitted and peeled
- ½ teaspoon spirulina and 1 tablespoon hemp seeds

Directions:

1. In a blender, combine all the ingredients and blend until smooth.
2. Serve immediately or store in the freezer in a resalable jar.

Nutrition value per serving: Calories: 431 Total fat: 16 g Carbohydrates: 70 g Fiber: 17 g

Protein: 13 g Calcium: 67% Vitamin D: 25% Vitamin B12: 31% Iron: 41% Zinc: 15%

Tropical Bliss Smoothie

Prep & Cooking time: 15 minutes   Servings: 1

Ingredients:

- 2 cups frozen pineapple and 1 banana
- 1¼ cup unsweetened coconut milk
- ¼ cup frozen coconut pieces and ½ teaspoon ground flaxseed
- 1 teaspoon hemp seeds

Directions:

1. In a blender, combine all the ingredients and blend until smooth.
2. Serve immediately or store in the freezer in a resalable jar.

Nutrition value per serving: Calories: 396 Total fat: 14 g Carbohydrates: 71 g Fiber: 11 g

Protein: 6 g Calcium: 64% Vitamin D: 31% Vitamin B12: 3% Iron: 19% Zinc: 7%

Very Berry Antioxidant Smoothie

Prep & Cooking time: 25 minutes   Servings: 1

Ingredients:

- 1 banana
- 1¼ cup unsweetened plant-based milk
- ½ cup frozen strawberries
- ½ cup frozen blueberries
- ½ cup frozen raspberries
- 3 pitted Medjool dates
- 1 tablespoon hulled hemp seeds
- ½ tablespoon ground flaxseed
- 1 teaspoon ground chia seeds **Directions**:

1. In a blender, combine all the ingredients and blend until smooth.
2. Serve immediately or store in the freezer in a resalable jar.

Nutrition value per serving: Calories: 538 Total fat: 11 g Carbohydrates: 111 g Fiber: 21 g

Protein: 10 g Calcium: 75% Vitamin D: 31% Vitamin B12: 8% Iron: *26%* Zinc: 13%

Easy Overnight Oats

Prep & Cooking time: 5 minutes, plus overnight Servings: 1

Ingredients:

- ½ cup rolled oats (check the label for gluten-free)
- ½ cup unsweetened plant-based milk
- 1 tablespoon nut butter
- ½ tablespoon cacao powder
- ½ teaspoon hulled hemp hearts
- ½ teaspoon maple
syrup Optional toppings:
- Dark chocolate chips
- Pecans
- Strawberries

Directions:

1. Combine all the ingredients in a mason jar or reusable food storage container.

2. Stir together, seal the lid, and place in the refrigerator overnight.
3. When ready to eat, add your favourite toppings.

Nutrition per serving: Calories: 347 Total fat: 14 g Carbohydrates: 48 g Fiber: 11 g

Protein: 12 g Calcium: 26% Vitamin D: 13% Vitamin B12: 1% Iron: 19% Zinc: 7%

Apple-Cinnamon Quinoa

Prep & Cooking time: 10 minutes   Servings: 1

Ingredients:

- 1½ cup of water
- 1½ cup diced Granny Smith apples
- ½ cup quinoa, rinsed
- 1 teaspoon ground flaxseed
- ½ teaspoon ground cinnamon

Optional toppings:
- Maple syrup and Nuts and seeds
- Nut butter and Fresh fruit
- Unsweetened plant-based milk

Directions:

1. In a medium pot over medium-high heat, combine the water, apples, quinoa, and flaxseed for 5 minutes or until the water has been fully absorbed.
2. Transfer the quinoa mixture to a bowl and stir in the cinnamon. Serve immediately as it is or with your favourite toppings.

Nutrition value per serving: Calories: 456 Total fat: 7 g Carbohydrates: 90 g Fiber: 12 g

Protein: 13 g Calcium: 7% Vitamin D: 0% Vitamin B12: 0% Iron: 29% Zinc: 1%

Strawberry-Kiwi Chia Pudding

Prep & Cooking time: 5 minutes, plus 4 hours   Servings: 2

Ingredients:

- 2   cups unsweetened coconut milk, divided
- 3   Medjool dates, pitted
- 1   tablespoon vanilla extract and ½ cup chia seedsToppings:
- 2   kiwis, sliced and 4 strawberries, sliced
- 2 tablespoons unsweetened coconut shreds
- 2 tablespoons sliced or chopped almonds

Directions:

1. In a food processor, blend ¾ cup of coconut milk, the dates, and vanilla. Pour the blended mix into a large reusable container or Mason jar.
2. Add the remaining 1¼ cups of coconut milk and the chia seeds. Cover the container and shake gently or stir to mix.
3. Store in the refrigerator overnight or for at least 4 hours until the chia seeds absorb all the milk. (Optional: stir once or twice as it is setting to avoid clumps.)
4. When ready to eat, top the pudding with kiwi, strawberries, coconut, and almonds. Store in the refrigerator for up to 5 days.

Nutrition per serving: Calories: 783 Total fat: 38 g Carbohydrates: 79 g Fiber: 48 g Protein: 27 g Calcium: 89% Vitamin D: 60% Vitamin B12: 100% Iron: 54% Zinc: 11%

Banana Protein Pancakes

Prep & Cooking time: 20 minutes   Servings: 2

Ingredients:

- 1½ cup unsweetened plant-based milk
- 1   cup quick oats and 1 banana
- ½ cup vital wheat gluten and ½ cup whole wheat flour
- 2   tablespoons maple syrup and 2 teaspoons vanilla extract
- 1 teaspoon pink Himalayan salt

Optional toppings:
- Sliced bananas and Pecans
- Hulled hemp seeds and Maple syrup

Directions:

1. In a food processor, combine all the ingredients except the optional toppings and mix until smooth. Use a ¼-cup measuring cup to pour ⅙ of the batter into a non-stick skillet over medium heat.
2. Once the edges of the pancake start to brown and bubble, flip and cook the other side. Repeat with the remaining batter. Serve immediately with your favorite toppings (if using) or store the pancakes in the refrigerator in a sealed container for up to 3 days.

Nutrition value per serving: Calories: 546 Total fat: 6 g Carbohydrates: 86 g
Fiber: 11 g Protein: 36 g Calcium: 42% Vitamin D: 23% Vitamin B12: 38% Iron: 34% Zinc: 11%

Blueberry Scones

Prep & Cooking time: 30 minutes, plus 20 minutes to freeze   Servings: 6

Ingredients:

- 2 cups whole wheat flour and ½ cup of coconut sugar
- 2½ teaspoons baking powder and ½ teaspoon pink Himalayan salt ½
- cup unsweetened applesauce and 3 tablespoons aquafaba (the liquid from a can of chickpeas)
- 2½ teaspoons vanilla extract and ⅓ Cup chopped almonds
- 1 cup fresh blueberries

Directions:

1. Preheat the oven to 400°F. In a large bowl, mix the flour, coconut sugar, baking powder, and salt. Add the applesauce, aquafaba, and vanilla and mix the dough together by hand. Gently stir in the almonds and blueberries.
2. Line an 8-inch square baking pan with parchment paper and spread the dough evenly in the pan. Freeze the dough for 20 minutes.
3. Bake for 25 minutes, or until light brown. Once cooled, cut into 6 scones. Store at room temperature in a covered container for up to 5 days.

Nutrition value per serving: Calories: 265 Total fat: 3 g Carbohydrates: 54 g
Fiber: 7 g Protein: 5 g Calcium: 16% Vitamin D: 0% Vitamin B12: 0%
Iron: 14% Zinc: 1%

Cinnamon French Toast

Prep & Cooking time: 15 minutes   Servings: 2

Ingredients:

- 1 cup unsweetened plant-based milk and ¾ cups firm tofu
- ½ teaspoon vanilla extract and ½ teaspoon ground cinnamon
- ¼ teaspoon ground flaxseed and 4 slices thick whole wheat bread

Directions:

1. In a blender, blend the milk, tofu, vanilla, cinnamon, and flaxseed until smooth.
2. Pour the mixture into a wide bowl.
3. Dip the bread slices into the mixture until evenly coated on both sides.
4. In a medium non-stick pan over medium heat, cook the bread slices, flipping when the bottom is light brown. Flip again, if needed.

Nutritional value per serving Calories: 642 Total fat: 20 g Carbohydrates: 92 g Fiber: 14 g

Protein: 31 g Calcium: 230% Vitamin D: 25% Vitamin B12: 0% Iron: 40% Zinc: 38%

Chapter 18: Cooking Tips

Tips for a Fast Day Cooking

1. Increase the measure of low-calorie: Green vegetables are hard to eat and ought to be bought somewhat before if huge amounts are required. Pan-seared vegetables are delectable. It is ideal for steaming delicately. Put resources into a layered bamboo liner to advance the well-being and cook protein and vegetables at different stages that are harmless to the ecosystem.

2. A few vegetables will profit by cooking. However, different vegetables ought to be eaten crudely: Cooking certain vegetables, for example, carrots, spinach, mushrooms, asparagus, cabbage, and peppers, annihilates cell structure without obliterating nutrients, permitting them to ingest more food. Mandolin makes the planning of crude vegetables brisk and simple.

3. Fasting days ought to be low in fat and not without fat: A teaspoon of olive oil can be utilized for cooking or sprinkled on vegetables to add flavour. Or, on the other hand, utilize a palatable oil splash to get a flimsy film. The arrangement incorporates greasy meats like nuts and pork. Add a light oil dressing to the plate of mixed greens. This implies that you are bound to ingest fat-solvent nutrients.

4. Lemon or orange dressing acids are said to assimilate more iron: From lavish greens, for example, spinach and kale. Watercress and orange are an extraordinary mix with few sesame seeds and sunflower seeds or whitening almonds scattered with a limited quantity of protein and crunch.

5. Cook in a container: To diminish unhealthy fats. On the off chance that the food sticks, sprinkle it with water.

6. Gauge the food after cooking: For an exact calorie check.

7. Dairy items are likewise included: Pick low-fat cheddar and skim milk, maintain a strategic distance from high-fat yoghurt, and pick a low-fat other option. Drop the latte and toss the margarine on a basic day. These are calorie traps.

8. Additionally, evade bland white starches: Like bread, potatoes, pasta; and rather, pick low GI carbs, for example, vegetables and gradually moving oats. Pick earthy-coloured rice and quinoa. Use cereal for breakfast longer than customary grains.

9. Ensure your fasting contains fibre: Eat apples and pears, have oats for breakfast, and add verdant vegetables.

10. On the off chance that conceivable, add flavours: Bean stew pieces kick a tasty dish. Balsamic vinegar gave causticity. We likewise add new spices—they are basically without calories; however, give the plate its character.

11. In the event that you eat protein, you stay longer: Stick to low-fat proteins, including a few nuts and vegetables. Eliminate meat skins and fats prior to cooking.

12. Soup on an eager day can be a hero: Particularly in the event that you pick a light soup with verdant greens (Vietnamese Pho is ideal, yet keep the noodles low). Soup is an incredible method to devour the fixings that you are tired of and that you battle inside the ice chest.

13. Whenever wanted, use agave as a sugar: Has lower GI.

Taste and Intermittent Fasting

This is a fragile issue for the vast majority, yet 7 days of planning ought to tackle it. That is the manner by which we are influenced by taste and need to ensure our taste buds. At first, the taste isn't simply fun. Inclination can pick the food you need, which is said to furnish nourishment with your body needs.

Taste implies craving, and hunger figures out what you eat. At the point when your body needs a specific supplement, it gives you a longing to search for and burn-through food sources that contain that supplement. It doesn't make any difference on the off chance that you are a veggie-lover that should not be taken lightly, yet in the event that you are new to veganism, you have a hunger for something that isn't on the menu.

The System Is as per the Following

At the point when you are a youngster, your folks will acquaint you with food sources that are important for your way of life and childhood. On the off chance that you are English, you get Bangers and Mash for breakfast. Mexicans get tortillas and quesadillas, and Americans call muesli and toast. It is the thing that you experienced childhood with (I realize it is considerably more than that—it is only a model).

At the point when you devour a specific arrangement of food sources, your body records and connects various nourishments with various encounters, for instance, on the off chance that you had sunflower seeds with grains in the first part of the day, your body will record the entirety of the sustenance you got from sunflower seeds by taking this nutrient E formula.

From that point on, when your body needs nutrient E, your body accidentally has a hunger for sunflower seeds. It gives you a craving for the flavour of sunflower seeds and the relationship it has in your mind between the requirement for nutrient E also, the inclination of sunflower seeds.

Taste is fundamental for our capacity to keep ourselves solid and renew what we need when we need it. It is important to ensure the nourishments we eat and not be happy with sweet-smelling food sources. Beginning an intermittent fasting way of life builds your feeling of taste and your longing for what you need, not what you are dependent on. It empowers you to tell them that the food they, for the most part, pine for isn't, at this point, accessible. Along these lines, we arranged the psyche and body of the main week to depend on taste as a guide for picking the nourishments on a case by case basis.

What's the significance here for you? Indeed, it saves you from eating pointless calories and putting on unnecessary weight. It works thusly. At the point when you need nutrient E from sunflower seeds, rather than picking regular sunflower seeds, you'll need to pick prepared and salted ones. Salt bids as I would prefer, and it makes propensities, yet the prepared grains are low in nutrient E, and to get the nutrient E, I take more seeds to compensate for the lack. This prompts more fatty admission and gives me pointless additional weight.

Thus, aside from preparing and taste, in the event that you can pick the specific food wellspring of the supplements you need is the taste. You can locate the most regular one you can find in these 7 days of readiness and until the 7 days of the housewarming. Picking nourishments will be spotless, and your craving will precisely reflect what your body needs to recharge.

Recall that intermittent fasting is a way of life change that we must be utilized to. Along these lines, don't think about this as a diet, and 7 days can't take you back to your old way of life. This is an adjustment in the essential perspective on and understanding the faculties. It is the immediate method to utilize your common fat-consuming cycle. It is the characteristic manner by which the human body develops.

Chapter 19: Frequently Asked Questions (FAQS)

Most sorts of changes accompany a ton of inquiries; intermittent fasting is the same. Here are some much of the time posed inquiries from fledgelings:

1. Would It Be a Good Idea for Me to Plan My Taking Care of and FastingTimes on the off Chance That I Work for the Time Being or Long Moves? Timetable your taking care of and fasting window as per your own time, which implies your taking care of window would be all the more so nights and overnight and the fasting a greater amount of the daytime when you are dozing.

2. Would I Be Able to Have Espresso? Indeed, you can have dark espressos,water, and plain soaks tea.

3. Would I Be Able to Add Cream/Sugar/Milk to My Espresso?

The objective of fasting isn't to add calories, so the appropriate response is no; you ought not to add anything to your espresso. Notwithstanding, I have known about cases in which intermittent fasters add under 50 calories to their espresso. They have professed to in any case be fruitful with intermittent fasting; I have heard that it doesn't influence their fasted state, yet remember all people are not made equivalent. I would not prescribe adding anything to your espresso, however, adding something to your espresso actually causes this a decent chance for the objective you have for yourself; at that point check it out.

4. Does Intermittent Fasting Function Admirably With Veganism, Paleo,Keto, Vegetarianism, or Some Other Styles of Eating?

Truly, the magnificence of intermittent fasting is that it tends to be joined with any way of eating except if, in any case, coordinated by a clinical expert. You can transform your way of eating into the 16:8 technique effortlessly, as this change doesn't confine or express the style/sorts of food you eat; it is explicitly founded on the circumstance of your eating.

5. Is There an Option in Contrast to the 16:8 Technique in the Event That ICan't at First Fast 16 Hours and Need to Move Gradually Up to 16?

Indeed, particularly for ladies, it is suggested that if ladies can't or are not able to do a 16 hour fast, they can begin with a 14-hour fasting window and a 10-hour taking care of window. This is suggested for ladies; however, men can begin here if necessary. When the 14 hours are dominated, you would then be able to move gradually up to the 16:8 strategy.

6. Would I Be Able to Have a Cheat Feast?

You can actually eat what you need when intermittent fasting; there are no nutrition-type limitations. There is no cheat feast to have except if you have concluded that you have put yourself on some prohibitive dinners/nourishments to not enjoy; assuming this is the case, at that point truly, yet I prescribe to consistently eat with some restraint.

7. What Are Some Solid Nibble Nourishments to Eat in a Hurry During MyTaking Care Window?

Pepperoni cuts, natural product, veggie plate, Skinny Pop popcorn singular sacks (except if you will consistently quantify the servings prior to devouring), turkey/hamburger jerky, singular peanut butter cups, entire grain cereal, almond milk, eggs, rice cakes, nuts (singular packs), hummus, and that's just the beginning.

8. I'm Excessively Ravenous During My Fasting Window; How Would ItBe Advisable for Me to Respond?

Be patient, and trust that your body will adjust to this change. This may set aside some effort; for a few, it happens fast; for other people, it might require a week or somewhere in the vicinity, yet this relies upon how you were eating prior to beginning this way of life. As per Collier in 2013, your body is as yet changing in accordance with how it was working previously and is battling you to return to that way, as a great many people were eating all the more often and perhaps more suppers or snacks during the day.

Ultimately, you won't feel thusly. At last, you will adjust to your taking care of and fasting windows, and the inclination to eat or the prospect of starving will get milder and milder until it disappears.

9. For What Reason Am I Not Losing Fat Faster, as Others Are?

It is, without a doubt, a mix of not eating the proper bits at the point when you are eating, as well as not planning to eat the correct food decisions. Albeit fat and weight reduction can, in any case, occur, it's more regular and obvious when the fitting food decisions and bits are chosen and arranged.

10. How Might I Stay Full More?

Eat more fibre, and drink more water, stay hydrated.

11. Do I Need to Eat Low Carb?

No, you can eat what you need during your taking care window. I suggest eating proportionately and picking on better food choices. Rather than white bread, pick entire grain bread. Rather than white rice, pick earthy coloured rice. Rather than anything with high fructose corn syrup, scratch it off; rather than a canned organic product, eat new organic products.

12. Would It Be a Good Idea for Me to Practice in the Fasted State?

You can, although it isn't needed. It is likewise not suggested on hard workdays. Imagine a scenario where I am on prescriptions and should eat with my morning meds. For this situation, you would have to make you take care of the window starts at whatever time you take your prescriptions. I would suggest accepting your medications as late as possible in the mornings yet get the approval of your arrangement from a clinical expert.

13. Would It Be a Good Idea for Me to Talk About This With My ClinicalExpert Prior to Starting the Change?

Truly, you ought to consistently talk about diet changes with a clinical expert before you start.

14. For What Reason Would It Be Advisable for One to Begin IntermittentFasting?

The main purpose behind beginning this diet plan is to get thinner without changing one's diet to an extraordinary level. With this diet plan, you are allowed to hold your body's bulk and stay fit. This is conceivable supposing that diminishes tummy fat as the diet advances. As this diet plan requires close to nothing change and no muddled schedules, it is a powerful and straightforward approach to get more fit.

15. Is Skipping Breakfast Thought About Undesirable for the Body?

No. This is a legend that the vast majority consider as being valid. This generalization should be maintained a strategic distance from. Some say that getting up and eating assists the body with getting the energy it needs for the entire day. That may be valid, yet on the off chance that you are following a solid diet for the remainder of your suppers, skipping breakfast ought not to influence your way of life. It may require some investment to become accustomed to avoiding a feast after you awaken with a vacant stomach; however, that will help the absorptive state occur to detoxify the body and clean your inner parts.

16. Is It all right to Take Supplements With an Intermittent Fasting Routine?

Truly, you can devour those also. Notwithstanding, you may have to beware of specific enhancements. Some of them may work in a way that is better than others. For example, fat-solvent nutrients will be more successful with your dinners during eating hours. Pick them over different sorts of enhancements.

A few specialists suggest burning-through BCAAs (stretched chain amino acids) prior to working out while fasting. Thusly, the body stays in a fasting state yet gets the protein to have a vivacious exercise schedule. It guarantees that you have high endurance and energy to turn out for a more drawn-out length without wearing out.

17. Will Intermittent Fasting Influence One's Digestion?

No, it won't influence the digestion if the fasting time frame is the present moment. In any case, examines have indicated that fasting for longer timeframes (like a few days) can diminish digestion. Intermittent fasting centres on transient fasting objectives, so it ought not to be terrible for digestion. All things being equal, it will support it for more viable handling.

18. Could a Kid Fast?

No, it would be an ill-conceived notion for a youngster to fast. Skipping breakfast can cause an absence of development hormones in a kid's body, and the person in question may not grow ordinarily. The kid may likewise need appropriate cerebrum work in the event that the individual follows intermittent fasting for a drawn-out period.

Conclusion

Intermittent Fasting is a diet that is simple and safe and makes dieting enjoyable. Although it contradicts a lot of today's views and ideas, there is science behind it. With all these new ideas and diets, you would think the world would be getting more fit instead of the obesity rate coming to an alltime high. Studies and science show Intermittent Fasting works, and if the Romans, the peak of fitness, used it to stay fit, why shouldn't we. Here are a few reasons why Intermittent fasting is not as insane as you think it is.

First, fasting has been practiced by diverse religious groups for decades. The health benefits of fasting for thousands of years have also been recognized by medical practitioners. Fasting is not some modern fad or a crazy marketing ploy. It's been around for a long time, and it works.

Second, fasting seems alien for many of us simply because no one speaks about it that much. The reason for this is that nobody stands to make much money by asking you not to eat their products, not to take their vitamins, or not to buy their goods. In other words, fasting is not a very marketable subject, and hence you are not very much subjected to advertising and marketing on it. The result is that it seems very strange or extreme, even though it really isn't,

Third, you've probably been fasting several times already, even though you don't realize it. Did you ever sleep late on the weekends and have a late brunch after that? Some individuals do every weekend. In circumstances such as these, we sometimes eat dinner the night before and then doesn't eat until 11 am or noon or even later. There is your 16–hour fast, and you didn't even think about it.

Finally, even if you do not plan to do intermittent fasting daily, I recommend doing one 24-hour fast. It's good to teach yourself that you'll survive just fine without food for a day. Intermittent fasting is a smart way to lose weight, replenish your cells, and probably add to your existence. However, intermittent fasting isn't for everybody. Well-being ultimately involves eating healthy foods, getting enough sleep, reducing stress, and achieving the right equilibrium.

Now you understand what intermittent fasting is and how it can help you lose weight efficiently, safely, and comfortably.

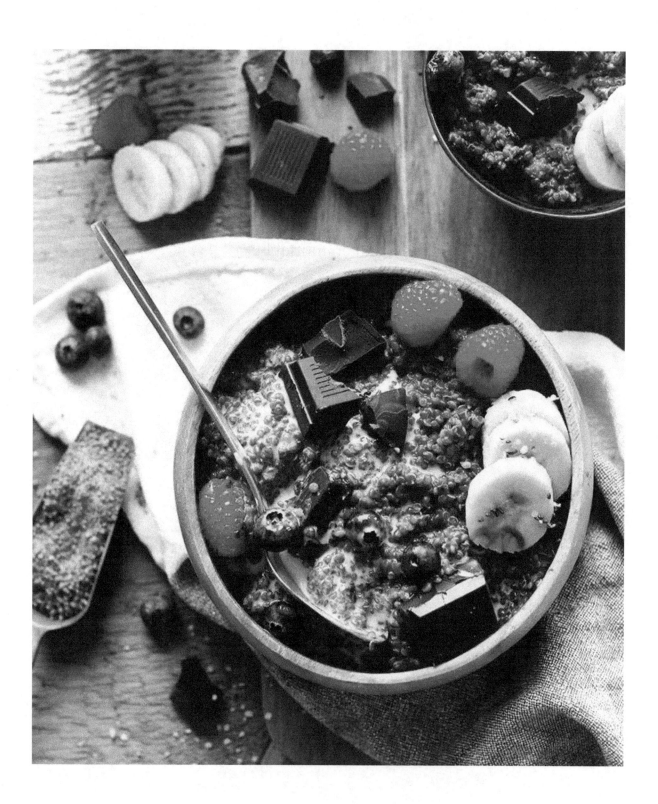

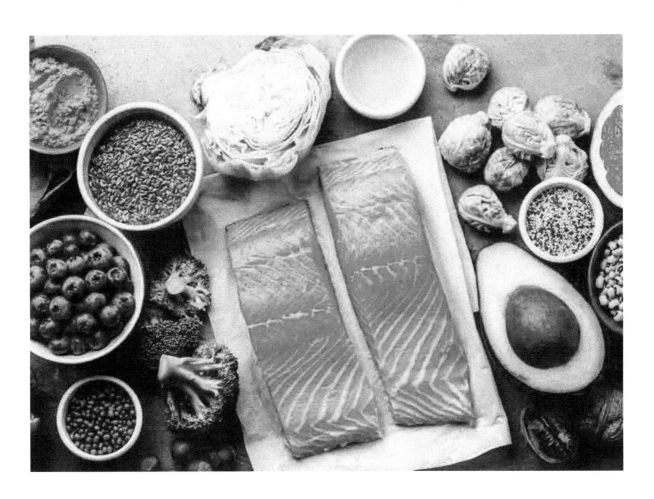

Study	Study population	Study design	Assessment tool	Study setting	Findings	Study details
Bogdan et al[27]	10 healthy male volunteers (age: 32–40 years) Location: France	Case crossover study with repeated measures	Blood samples were obtained every 4 hours, omitting the 02:00 time point, before and on the 23rd day of Ramadan	Free-living environment Controlled for meal timing and composition Did not control for light exposure, sleep schedule, or social habits that accompany Ramadan	A decreased and delayed night peak and a flattened slope of serum melatonin concentration in Ramadan	Volunteers slept 1 hour less during Ramadan than before Ramadan Melatonin concentrations were not measured late at night, which fails to address the possibility of a late peak in melatonin concentration
BaHammam et al[30]	8 healthy young adults (age: 31.8±2 years) Location: Saudi Arabia	Case crossover study with repeated measures	Saliva samples were collected at three time points over a 24-hour period (08:00, 16:00, and 00:00) before and on the 7th and 21st days of Ramadan	In-laboratory monitoring Controlled for meal timing and composition Controlled for sleep duration Did not control for light exposure or social habits that accompany Ramadan	A significant decrease in melatonin concentrations at 00:00 and 16:00 during Ramadan Melatonin profiles continued to show the same trend during Ramadan, but with a flatter slope	Melatonin concentrations were not measured late at night, which fails to address the possibility of a late peak in melatonin concentration
Almeneessier et al[28]	8 healthy young adults (age: 26.6±4.9 years) Location: Saudi Arabia	Case crossover study with repeated measures	Blood samples were collected at 22:00, 02:00, 04:00, 06:00, and 11:00 before Ramadan and while performing fasting outside Ramadan month and on the second week of Ramadan	In-laboratory monitoring Controlled for light exposure, sleep schedule, sleep duration, energy expenditure, and meal composition	Intermittent fasting during Ramadan has no significant effect on the circadian pattern of melatonin	Assessed melatonin level when volunteers were fasting outside Ramadan month to control for lifestyle changes that accompany Ramadan

CPSIA information can be obtained
at www.ICGtesting.com
Printed in the USA
BVHW061953080621
609008BV00008B/1827